T0256965

Is the 'baby boom generation' more or less healthy than previous generations? What will be the impact of this aging population on the Canadian health care system? In response to these questions, *Baby Boomer Health Dynamics* looks at the health status of a generation that makes up over one-third of the Canadian population – the largest segment of society – with the leading edge reaching their sixty-fifth birthday in 2011 and their eighty-fifth by 2031. This study presents national data spanning twenty-two years, which are analysed, assessed, and integrated with current knowledge about the health of Canadians.

In *Baby Boomer Health Dynamics*, Andrew Wister argues that the health of a population is affected by experiences of cohorts as they form unique health and illness trajectories connected to their size, composition, earlier life experiences, and exposure to historical events. A cohort analysis of major national Canadian surveys collected between 1978–9 and 2000–1 constitutes the core of the primary research. In addition to a discussion of general population trends, the author provides comparisons of the baby boom generation with the previous generation, and looks at the influence of such factors as socioeconomic status, regional differences, and foreign-born status on lifestyle behaviours. Focusing on four health behaviours that have been proven to be major risk factors for disease – smoking, unhealthy exercise, obesity, and heavy drinking – Wister explores the long-term implications of key lifestyle-health issues, notably the concurrent trends over the last two decades of increased exercise levels and a significant rise in obesity. This paradox raises questions about the eating habits of North Americans, particularly in regard to fast food consumption.

Providing a wealth of data and insightful analysis of issues and trends, *Baby Boomer Health Dynamics* is essential reading for students and practitioners in the fields of sociology, demography, gerontology, epidemiology, and health sciences.

ANDREW V. WISTER is chair of the Department of Gerontology at Simon Fraser University.

Baby Boomer Health Dynamics

How Are We Aging?

Andrew V. Wister

UNIVERSITY OF TORONTO PRESS
Toronto Buffalo London

© University of Toronto Press Incorporated 2005
Toronto Buffalo London
Printed in Canada

ISBN 0-8020-8957-7 (cloth)
ISBN 0-8020-8635-7 (paper)

Printed on acid-free paper

Library and Archives Canada Cataloguing in Publication

Wister, Andrew V., 1955–
    Baby boomer health dynamics : how are we aging? / Andrew V.
Wister.

    Includes bibliographical references and index.
    ISBN 0-8020-8957-7 (bound).   ISBN 0-8020-8635-7 (pbk.)

    1. Baby boom generation – Health and hygiene – Canada.   2. Middle
aged persons – Health and hygiene – Canada.   3. Health behavior – Age
factors – Canada.   4. Health status indicators – Canada.   I. Title.

RA408.B33W58 2005   614.4′2′08440971   C2004-905883-5

University of Toronto Press acknowledges the financial assistance to its publishing program of the Canada Council for the Arts and the Ontario Arts Council.

University of Toronto Press acknowledges the financial support for its publishing activities of the Government of Canada through the Book Publishing Industry Development Program (BPIDP).

Contents

Tables and Figures

Tables

Appendix

Figures

Appendix

Preface

This book was written in response to the mounting interest in population health in Canada, and, in particular, concerns that the baby boom generation will place an enormous burden on the health care system. The main objective of this book is therefore to examine the population health dynamics of the baby boom generation by integrating a review of selected literature and original research. A primary focus is on a selection of health behaviours that are major risk factors for disease: smoking, unhealthy exercise, obesity, and heavy drinking. The recent declaration that we are experiencing an obesity crisis, and, moreover, that obesity is the 'new tobacco,' emphasize the need for elucidating the health characteristics of major target groups of Canadians. Key questions guiding this book include: (1) Are the baby boomers healthier or unhealthier than previous generations? and (2) What are the implications of these patterns for the Canadian health care system? Current knowledge in this field is sparse and fraught with stereotypical images rather than fact. Some researchers paint 'boomers' as individuals who are healthier and wealthier than prior generations, whereas others maintain that they have a 'poor health report card' because they are prone to obesity and chronic illness, and, therefore, will break the public purse when they become the elderly of tomorrow. These questions are fundamental to the future of Canadian society, given the relative size and placement of the baby boomers in the population structure. Baby boomers comprise approximately one-third of the population concentrated in a 20-year span, defined here as persons born between 1946 and 1965, and, moreover, they are moving up the age escalator to the top floors. Indeed, those in the leading edge of the baby boom generation will reach their 65th birthdays in 2011, and by 2031 baby boomers will range in age between 65 and 85.

The unique research in *Baby Boomer Health Dynamics* includes a detailed health profiling and cohort analyses of data from a selection of major national

Canadian health surveys between 1978/79 and 2000/2001 – a 22-year period. Age-sex-specific health profiles of the baby boom and adjacent cohorts are presented for the major lifestyle risk factors, major chronic illnesses, and doctor visits. *Intra-* and *inter*-comparisons of all available five-year age-sex cohorts spanning the lifecycle of Canadians are conducted in order to identify past, current, and future patterns and their implications for society. Separate chapters deal explicitly with comparisons of the baby boom generation of today with individuals of similar ages over the previous two-plus decades. In addition, two 10-year age cohorts comprising the 20-year baby boom generation (younger and older boomers) are compared and contrasted for the purpose of detailing heterogeneity within this generation. The influence of socioeconomic status (income and education), region, and foreign-born status on healthy lifestyle trends is also assessed.

The theoretical basis for research into the population health dynamics of baby boomers draws from the Social Change Model developed by Riley (1993). Based on this framework, the health of a population can be understood as a combination of cohorts with unique health and illness trajectories connected to their size, composition, earlier life experiences, and exposure to differing normative milieu and historical events. It therefore integrates elements of age stratification, life course, and cohort approaches to aging and health. The age stratification approach concentrates on the ways in which a population is age-segregated. The life course approach traces characteristics of the lives of a single cohort or generation of individuals (i.e., baby boomers) over their lifetime and adds the notion of human agency – the proactive role that the individual plays in shaping social structure. Additionally, the cohort approach studies characteristics of two or more successive birth cohorts, and therefore melds both cross-sectional and life course patterns of health and disease. Other major theories that have a bearing on health behaviours are also integrated within a transdisciplinary framework in an effort to better understand how aging processes at individual and population levels interact to affect population health.

Baby Boomer Health Dynamics specifically addresses a number of questions and issues that have attracted the attention of researchers, policy-makers, and health care organizations. For example, what are the most important health trajectories of the baby boom generation? Furthermore, how will they influence future patterns of health status and health utilization across major social categories, such as gender, education, income, region, and foreign-born status? And do macro shifts in the economy or in population education levels affect lifestyle behaviours, health status indicators, or self-reported health utilization of these persons? In so doing, this volume explicates several key lifestyle-health conundrums that are revealed in the analysis and discussed in the latter chapters of the book. For instance, there is an apparent paradox in the concurrent population trends of increasing exercise levels and a significant rise in obesity over the last few decades. In order to explain these disconnecting patterns, changes in leisure-time physical activity, work-related activity, eating habits, fast food super-sizing, and environmental factors influencing healthy lifestyles are investigated. The final sections of the book also shed light on the question: What will elderly baby boomers be like in terms of health and health care utilization? This discussion is placed within the context of health programming and health care reform in Canada.

Acknowledgments

Foremost, I wish to thank my wife Barbara and my daughter Kayzia for their continual support and patience throughout the various stages of development of this book. I am also appreciative of my parents for their encouragement of my academic pursuits. I recognize as well the assistance of my research assistant, Mary Rogers, who helped make the presentation of complex data clear, accurate, and readable. Additionally, I am grateful for the statistical support from a fellow wine connoisseur, Doug Talling. This volume also benefited from the editorial wisdom of Stephen Kotowych, Anne Laughlin, and Patricia Thorvaldson at the University of Toronto Press. My mentor, Dr. Thomas Burch, had a significant influence on my development as an academic and as a person, for which I am indebted. Finally, the ideas of Matilda White Riley need to be recognized as a key foundation to the work comprising this book.

BABY BOOMER HEALTH DYNAMICS

1

The Baby Boomer Phenomenon

Who Are the Baby Boomers?

Understanding current and future patterns of population health of Canadians necessitates consideration of the 'baby boom generation,' given its size and placement within the age structure. The cohorts that comprise the baby boom are the largest in Canadian history, and those in the leading one are anticipated to reach their 60th birthday in 2006, their 65th by the year 2011, and their 75th in 2021. By 2031, the full 'boomer' generation will be over the age of 65, and the front cohort will have turned 85. While many stereotypes persist concerning the characteristics of baby boomers that are present in both popular and academic literature, details of the health of these persons is limited, especially transformations in health status that have occurred as this generation moves through middle age and into the years designating older adulthood.

In order to study the baby boom generation, it is first useful to define the concept of 'generation.' Although several definitions of what constitutes a generation exist, for the purpose of this research the term is delineated using three principal characteristics: (1) a generation comprises a set of individual birth cohorts (each typically viewed as an individual year of birth unless grouped into a larger cohort); (2) it tends to include enough individual birth cohorts to separate children and parents – approximately 20 to 30 years; and (3) a generation typically exhibits characteristics or 'watersheds' that distinguish it from other generations related to the size and composition of the cohorts from which it is comprised, and the attributes of these individuals (Morgan, 1998a). Thus, while cohorts are distinguishable in terms of year of birth, generations are marked by a combination of distinctive cultural values, attitudes, or compositional elements (i.e., relative size) that set them apart from other generations. It is also understood that generations need to be studied in terms of age, cohort, and historical period, as well as their interactions (Giele and Elder, 1998). The age at which individuals of a particular birth cohort (age effects) – those who share social experiences at the same point in life as their age peers (cohort effects) – are exposed to particular historical events (period effects) will define a generation. In North America the large birth cohorts of the baby boom transitioned from the teenage years into young adulthood during the turbulent 1960s and 1970s, which distinguish them from earlier generations in significant ways. During their teenage and young adult years, baby boomers reacted against the values held by their parent's generation, formed in the 1940s and 1950s, choosing instead to embrace a spirit of individualism and freedom of behaviour that included experimentation with drugs, sex, and new forms of music and art. They also reacted against the Vietnam War, racism, sexism, consumerism, and other mainstream socio-political forces and normative structures in society. Setting them apart from other generations (e.g., the beat generation of the 40s and 50s) was also the fact that the baby boomers were considerably larger in sheer numbers. As stated by Owram (1999:210), 'This was, after all, "the" generation, and the sense of being involved in a vast peer-group revolution was very very powerful.'

There are several common, age-related definitions of the baby boom generation. Denton and Spencer (1997) define them using the narrowest range, a 15-year period comprising persons born between 1946 and 1960. According to Cole and Castellano (1996), the baby boom is defined as the generation of persons born between 1946 and 1964, during which time birth cohorts increased dramatically in size compared to previous decades. This was primarily the result of two converging trends: a rise in the post-Second World War marriage rate, and families having more children closer together. In his popular 1996 book, *Boom, Bust, and Echo: How to Profit from the Coming Demographic Shift*, David Foot focuses on three main generations: (1) baby boomers, which he defines as Canadians born during the 20-year period between 1947 and 1966; (2) the baby bust generation, which includes those born between 1967 and 1979; and (3) the baby boom echo generation, which includes many of the children of the baby boom generation – persons born between 1980 and 1995. Furthermore, the back end of the baby boom generation, about 2.6 million persons born between 1960 and 1966, are in their early to mid-30s and have been labelled Generation X (Foot, 1996).

Since the birth cohorts of the early 1960s are particularly large proportionate to the post-Second World War period, a 20-year definition will be adopted for this study: persons born between 1946 and 1965. Diverging slightly from Foot (1996), however, we employ the more traditional starting point of the post-war birth cohort of 1946 and include all cohorts up to and including 1965.

This 20-year period more accurately reflects the bulging birth cohorts that continued into the early '60s, and allows for equal division of this generation into two, 10-year birth cohorts that can be considered to represent *younger* and *older* baby boomers, respectively. We also divide baby boomers into four 5-year cohorts suitable for *inter-* and *intra-cohort* comparative analyses. Since a consensus is lacking in the literature as to whether the baby boomers actually comprise a single homogeneous generation (Morgan, 1998a), the exploration of the health dynamics of younger and older baby boomers appears to be warranted and may be useful in distinguishing distinctive characteristics within the baby boom generation. However, for the purpose of the present discussion, we will refer to the baby boomers as a singular generation, albeit one that is not assumed to be homogeneous in terms of important economic, social, and demographic markers. For example, although we assume people of a particular age are members of the baby boom generation, in fact, a significant proportion of these individuals may have immigrated to Canada and are not baby boomers in a cultural sense. Thus, we will also need to examine educational, income, regional, and, in particular, foreign-born status elements of baby boomer health dynamics.

Baby boomers comprise a significant segment of the Canadian population. Based on the 2001 Canadian census, there were 9.4 million (9,405,055) persons born between 1946 and 1965, a remarkable 31.3% of the total enumerated Canadian population of 30,007,095. These individuals would have been aged 36 to 55 in 2001. If we separate our 20-year baby boom generation into two 10-year groups, it can be observed that 5.1 million (5,128,380) persons, or 54.5% of all boomers, are 'younger boomers' born between 1956 and 1965. In addition, approximately 4.3 million (4,276,675) individuals, or 45.5% of all boomers, are 'older boomers' born between 1946 and 1955. Thus, younger boomers comprise a slightly bigger proportion of this generation. If we examine the 2001 Canadian census data closer, we discover that the largest individual age cohort in the total population in that year entails persons aged 40 at that time (born in 1961), a total of 528,755 persons. This is followed by 525,550 persons aged 38 who were born in 1963; 522,755 individuals aged 41 who were born in 1960; and 518,635 persons aged 39 who were born in 1962. In comparison, there were only 391,440 Canadians in 2001 who were aged 29 (born in 1972), and only 288,110 persons aged 59 (born in 1942). Thus, the most populated age cohorts in 2001 were born between 1960 and 1963, and were aged 38 to 41 in 2001. These four age cohorts comprise about 2.1 million Canadians, almost 7% of the total population, and an amazing 22.3% of the baby boom generation born between 1946 and 1965. Note that these four largest age cohorts in 2001 are not identical to the largest birth cohorts, since their size is influenced by mortality and immigration trends between the date of birth and the census year 2001.

Baby Boomers and Population Aging

As can be observed in Figure 1.1, the baby boomers form a noticeable bulge in the population age structure of Canada. In this figure, the protruding baby boom generation is shown for 1981, 2001 and 2006 with males and females displayed separately on each side of this 'age pyramid.' Also note that the 'echo effect' of the baby boomers can be seen in the 2006 scenario, which is the smaller bulge representing the children of the baby boom generation. Obvious from this figure is the fact that, as time passes, the baby boomers are gradually moving up the age structure (metaphorically described as the 'pig in the python'), and are fast approaching their elder years. The front edge of the baby boomers (born in 1946) will be 60 years of age in 2006, and 65 in 2011. But the full 'gerontological impact' of this generation on health care will probably not be felt at least until the point at which the last cohort of the baby boomers becomes 65 in 2031, at which time the front cohort will be age 85. Indeed, the percentage of the total Canadian population aged 65 and over has increased slowly for the last several decades, but will obviously gain momentum as the baby boomers move through the top of the age pyramid. For instance, the proportion of Canadians aged 65 and over was 7.6% in 1961, 8.1% in 1971, 9.7% in 1981, 11.6% in 1991, and 13% in 2001 (Statistics Canada, 2001a). However, this rate has been estimated to reach 14.5% in 2011, 18.9% in 2021, and 21.4% in 2026. Thus, population aging and the aging of the baby boomers are intertwined demographic patterns that have far-reaching consequences for society.

The Social Significance of Aging Baby Boomers

The social significance of the baby boom generation is that, as it ages, it will continue to account for at least one-third of the Canadian population, and since it is compressed into a 20-year range in the age structure, it will have a marked impact on the course of many key social, economic, and health trends. Indeed, the main thesis of Foot (1996) is that the relative size, characteristics, and behaviour of the baby boomers, in relation to other generations, will dictate most major consumer trends, including patterns of education enrolment and health care utilization, with the costs associated with the latter expected to skyrocket. He has also predicted that the market for detached homes will deflate once the baby boomers reach older ages and begin to downsize their

Figure 1.1 Age Pyramid of the Population of Canada, 1 July, 1981, 2001, and 2006

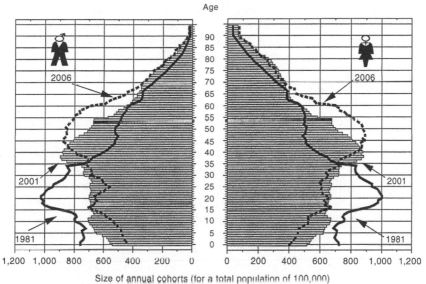

Source: Statistics Canada, Cat. 91-213, March 2002.

accommodations. Furthermore, Foot forecasts that bird watching and other leisure pursuits common among older adults will grow once the 'boomers' reach their golden years. However, these predictions have come under attack because they sometimes oversimplify complex phenomena by applying what has been termed 'demographic determinism' or 'apocalyptic demography' (Gee, 2000). As the latter term denotes, predictions of this nature often entail exaggeration of potential 'social problems' into 'crises' associated with particular demographic trends, such as rapid population aging. Dychtwald (1997:11), for instance, argues that American baby boomers will be faced with a number of such crises, including a pandemic of chronic disease, mass dementia, a care-giving crunch, conflict with other generations, and inadequate pensions. In fact, he states: 'When I look toward the future, I can clearly see a variety of train wrecks about to happen – *all of which are preventable*, but only if we fully understand the relationship between our current decisions and their future outcomes and only if we initiate corrective action *now*' (original emphasis).

One major criticism directed towards this approach to demographic analysis is that linear projections are typically put forth using selected population characteristics under the assumption that most behaviour can be explained using only demographic variables (Gee, 2000). For instance, Foot (1996) argues that two-thirds of all behaviour is explained through demographics, that is, the changing age structure. It is not uncommon for some researchers to select a current social trend that contains significant age-related differences, such as housing price, sales, type, tenure, or living arrangement, and to predict future patterns by applying population projections to that age rate. The obvious assumption is that, except for age compositional shifts, all other factors of influence remain approximately equal. For example, it would have to be assumed that social norms, values, and personal preferences underlying behaviour remain unchanged over the time period being projected. Yet, a plethora of sociological and social demographic studies have established demonstratively the salience of normative and preference structures in affecting a variety of social behaviours, and, moreover, that they are continually reshaping over time. Given the distinct values of the baby boom generation coupled with exposure to unique historical experiences, why would we expect them to follow the same health trajectories as their parents, except in larger numbers? Furthermore, the degree to which baby boomers will either be the cause of, or will face, various 'crises' is controversial. Thus, there are both theoretical and empirical reasons why making relatively simplistic linear demographic predictions of social behaviour based on this method, and portraying them as crises, is tenuous at best.

There is little doubt that the basic idea that cohort size and its compositional characteristics related to specific cohorts influence many social and economic trends, and that these elements also shape social policy. These types of projections have some use in identifying important social trends of the future, *assuming all else remains the same*. For instance, if age-specific rates of hospital use remain unchanged, then we can estimate the influence of the large birth cohorts of the late 1950s and early 1960s on future rates. However, the complexity of relationships among demographic, economic, and social factors also demands attention. Seminal research by Easterlin (1991, 1996) has provided empirical support for a cyclical pattern among the size of a birth cohort, employment opportunities, and economic prosperity. According to this thesis, large cohorts generate economic upswings once those persons reach their labour force years, which in turn result in higher fertility rates. Smaller birth cohorts have the opposite effect. Additionally, age-related patterns change over time because of shifting expectations, preferences, and attitudes, many of which are enveloped in age, period, and cohort processes. Clearly then, there is considerable non-linearity, complexity, and heterogeneity in the health dynamics of baby boomers, and that research is needed to explicate these patterns (Morgan, 1998a, 1998b).

Regardless of the arbitrary end point of the baby boom, Canada will continue to undergo significant population aging. The proportion of persons over the age of 65 will expand more rapidly as the baby boomers enter their elder years. As previously stated, according to the definition used here, the first age cohort (persons born in 1946) of the baby boom generation will turn 65 in 2011. In less than 30 years, by 2031, the full baby boom generation will be 65 years of age and over and the first cohort will be aged 85. Using the 'medium' or 'standard' population projections, the median age of the Canadian population will rise almost nine years between 1996 levels and 2031, to age 44.Thus, half of the population will be aged 44 and over. Moreover, the future population aged 65 and over will be about 2.5 times as large as it is now – 9.2 million compared to 3.7 million persons (Denton and Spencer, 1997). The aging of the baby boom generation is at the heart of these impressive trends in population aging, and it is not surprising that this phenomenon has become ubiquitous in forecasting key demographic, social, and economic trends, as well as precipitating discussions pertaining to the wider implications of these patterns for society (McDaniel, 1986).

It is, however, premature to assume that there is an imminent health care crisis, or pension crisis, for that matter, since the pace of population aging will not result in a rapid incline in the number of older adults over age 65 until multiple baby boomer age cohorts hit their golden years. Furthermore, it will be at least 20 years before the aging of the baby boom generation significantly influences health service utilization because of the obvious lag before they reach the age of 75 or over, at which point health needs rise more steeply (Denton and Spencer, 2000; Moore and Rosenberg, 1997). It is recognized, however, that this pattern could be exacerbated due to observed acceleration in the rates of health service utilization over the last few decades among specific age-sex groups, in particular, higher hospital and physician use among persons aged 75 and over (Barer, Evans, and Hertzman, 1995; Evans, McGrail, Morgan, Barer, and Hertzman, 2001). In question is whether the rise in health care utilization is a reflection of poorer health status of older adults over time or inflation in health care because of a growing supply and/or cost of doctors, health care technology, and other treatments. Barer et al. (1995) and Evans et al. (2001) have used the British Columbia-linked administrative data to analyse health utilization patterns over two decades and have clearly demonstrated significant elevation in the cost of pharmaceuticals, doctor-patient ratios, and hospital services, suggesting greater health care intensity targeting older adults.

Concurrently, consistent with Fries' (1983) prediction of a *compression of morbidity*, there is evidence that persons over 65 are experiencing the onset of disease later in life, and therefore this onset is compressed into a shorter time frame. Research shows that while life expectancy continues to rise, so does disability-free life expectancy (Manuel and Schultz, 2001; Robine, Mormiche, and Sermet, 1998), which is the number of years of remaining life that one can expect to live in reasonably good health or without being seriously disabled (Chappell, Gee, McDonald, and Stones, 2003; Robine et al., 1998). Thus, it would appear at first glance that important health status and health utilization trends are occurring that require careful analysis.

However, growth of the health care industry in conjunction with a population that lives longer free of major disability for increasingly longer periods does not provide a complete picture of what the future holds in store. Lifestyle risk factors (e.g., smoking, exercise, and diet) and the prevalence and incidence of chronic illnesses that occur as people age are constantly in flux, and they also require attention in our analyses of health status and health care forecasts. Indeed, the most accurate predictions will likely not mirror the present, but will reflect the dynamics and complexity that underlie social and individual change.

It is imperative, therefore, to set the stage for readjustments in the health policy arena in anticipation of shifting patterns of at least three major health domains: determinants of health, health status, and health service use (Blanchette and Valcour, 1998). Two major gaps in this literature are addressed in this book: (1) research that identifies significant shifts in major health patterns, including an elaboration of the relationships among them; and 2) detailed health profiles of age-sex-specific cohorts to expound the heterogeneity of the baby boom generation (Wister and Gutman, 1994).

Objectives and Primary Questions Guiding This Book

The main objective of this book is to examine the population health dynamics of the Canadian population generally, and the baby boom generation specifically, over approximately a 22-year period. One method of approaching this research is to use cohort analyses, which responds to limitations of cross-sectional and panel designs for studying aging processes across time (Schaie, 1965). This necessitates a detailed health profiling of age cohorts based on data from a selection of national Canadian health surveys between 1978/79 and 2000/2001, for which comparable data are available. Age-sex-specific health profiles of baby boomers and for the population as a whole are necessary in order to detail substantial health trends in society. Analysis of the total

Canadian population allows for an opportunity to place the baby boom generation within the emergent health patterns of the full population, and, additionally, lets us perform comparative cohort analyses. Additionally, population
health characteristics will be identified for the 20-year baby boom generation,
and compared across levels of education, income, region, and foreign-born
status, in order to focus the analysis on this important segment of the
population. Finally, the two 10-year age cohorts comprising the 20-year
baby boom generation (demarked as younger and older baby boomers) will
be compared and contrasted for the purpose of detailing heterogeneity within
that generation.

To date, Canadian national health studies have collected essential information on a considerable number of substantive areas associated with population
health, health promotion, individual health status, and health utilization. For
example, there is a plethora of research that has established the significance of
social determinants of both health behaviours and health status (i.e., factors
associated with poverty, age-related patterns, gender differences, etc.); differences in education, knowledge, and exposure to risk factors linked to the
health of Canadians (e.g., exercise, smoking, hypertension, cholesterol, and
weight); and associations between all of the above and utilization of health
services (Cockerham, Lueschen, Kunz, and Spaeth, 1986; Carrière and Pelletier,
1995; Health and Welfare Canada, 1988; Health Canada, 1993; Wister 1995,
1996). However, a review of the literature on population health clearly demonstrates that there are many areas in need of research activity. One of these is the
documentation of patterns and comparative analyses of lifestyle health
behaviours. Lifestyles are of central importance to population health
(McPherson, 2004). In fact, it has been estimated that behavioural risk factors
such as smoking, physical inactivity, poor diet, and their sequelae account for
approximately one-third of all deaths (McGinnis and Foege, 1993; Nawaz,
Adams, and Katz, 2000), and are directly or indirectly responsible for a
significant proportion of health care spending. The aim of this book is therefore to analyse lifestyle behaviours and other selected determinants of health,
as well as indicators of health status and health utilization among successive
cohorts of Canadians, with a focus on baby boomer trends.

The proposed analyses will shed light on a number of research questions
that have attracted and continue to attract the attention of researchers, policy-
makers, and health care organizations. For example, what are the most salient
age, period, and cohort patterns in the health trajectories of the baby boom
generation compared to previous ones? How do patterns in healthy lifestyles
differ across the selected socio-demographic determinants of health (i.e., age,
gender, education, income, region, and foreign-born status)? Do more edu-

cated boomers engage in higher levels of physical activity, and so on, and if so, has this changed over time? In addition, do persons who engage in and maintain healthy lifestyles have lower utilization rates of the formal health system over an extended period of time than persons who do not? Finally, do macro shifts in the economy, education levels of the population, or immigration trends modify lifestyle behaviours of persons belonging to different age cohorts – for example, those at the front end of the baby boom compared to those at the end?

2

Baby Boomers and Population Health

How Should We Study Baby Boomer Health Dynamics?

The theoretical basis for research into the population health dynamics of baby boomers draws from the Social Change Model developed by Riley (1993). This framework integrates principle elements of *age stratification, life course,* and *cohort* approaches to the study of population aging, and applies these concepts to the examination of population health (see McPherson, 2004, for a more complete discussion). Age-stratification of populations, at least in its earlier formulation, relies on cross-sectional information to understand age-related patterns of behaviour or strata at one point in time. It typically entails comparing age-related differences: for example, age patterns in the prevalence of diabetes. The life course approach traces characteristics of the lives of a single cohort of individuals (i.e., persons of the same birth cohort) over a significant period of their life (what is known as a life course) for the purpose of examining the causes and consequences of health. Earlier life experiences are assumed to have bearing on later ones, and individuals are assumed to interact with the creation of social structures through human agency (Marshall, 1999; Mitchell, 2003). For example, one might follow health trajectories of baby boomers as they move from young adulthood, to middle adulthood, and finally into mature adulthood. This would require trend analysis of several cross-sectional health surveys spanning the period of life under study for the baby boomer generation. The cohort approach focuses on health characteristics of two or more successive birth cohorts, and integrates both cross-sectional and life course patterns of health. In this case, a comparative analysis of health changes over the life courses of different birth cohorts (for example, younger and older baby boomers) would be conducted using a series of national health surveys. An essential feature of this perspective is that the study of aging-related patterns and their association with social structural change requires longitudinal analyses in order to reflect the dynamic nature of these relationships over time and place. Cohort analyses are at the fulcrum of this type of thinking. Although there are advantages in following the same individuals over time using a panel design, in Canada these data are only available for a short period beginning in the mid-1990s. The use of a series of cross-sectional surveys is a more common design in order to undertake cohort analyses.

According to Riley (1993), this approach has four major theoretical principles. *First*, the cohort approach affords an opportunity to identify mutable factors affecting health by juxtaposing cohorts of individuals who grow old under different historical circumstances, cohorts that can be examined in conjunction with gender, education, income, employment status, region, and other individual and environmental factors. As stated by Riley (1993:43), 'it has been clearly demonstrated that members of cohorts already old differ markedly from those cohorts not yet old in many critical respects that can influence health: diet, exercise, standard of living, education, work history, medical care, and experience with acute versus chronic diseases.' *Second*, age-relevant and irrelevant life course trends can be identified when historical period effects (such as the growth of the fast food industry, the AIDS epidemic, or economic recessions) either influence a whole population or are observed to affect only specific age groups. For example, Elder and Rockwell (1979) found that the Great Depression exerted more deleterious effects on younger cohorts of men than on the older ones in terms of future economic status because of their age when these events took place. *Third*, the cohort approach can improve forecasts of future health characteristics of people by identifying distinctive patterns among successive cohorts. If there is a clear pattern in cohort-related changes in health, then it is possible to predict population health characteristics with a certain degree of accuracy. And *fourth*, the health of a population can be understood best as a combination of cohorts with unique health and illness trajectories connected to their size, composition, earlier life experiences, and exposure to differing normative milieu and historical events (Riley, 1993).

Thus, the Social Change Model emphasises the reshaping of population health as successive cohorts transition through their life cycle, as well as the population age structure, as if on an upward bound escalator (Ryder, 1965). It can be added that the incline of the escalator represents health characteristics such as the prevalence of a chronic illness, and is constantly shifting due to relevant interrelationships among social and political change at the *macro-* and *micro*-level linked to cohorts and individuals. At the macro level, the cohorts moving along the age escalator are differentiated by their sizes, compositions, and historical experiences, such as the health care reform facing the baby boomers, the expansion of post-secondary education, the influence on this generation of Internet health information and globalization. At the micro level, individuals and groups of individuals (i.e., cohorts) make decisions about health behaviours and are exposed to varying life chances and opportunities connected to genetic, physiological, psychological, and social elements. For example, decisions to frequently eat fast food may determine levels of obesity and in some instances lead to diabetes. The *meso* or policy environment falls between the macro and micro levels. The government-sponsored anti-smoking legislation and related advertising is an example of the meso-level policy environment that bridges the other two. This approach therefore implores the researcher to investigate the age, period, and cohort effects associated with successive cohorts over time, and to develop a priori hypotheses about relationships among the three domains: macro (structural changes), meso (program and policy changes linking the two extremes), and micro (individual change) levels. For example, this approach might investigate hypotheses pertaining to the impact of educational or income-distribution changes in the population on healthy lifestyle behaviour; the influence of the well-known ParticipAction program on levels of physical activity in the population; or hypotheses about the growing sizes of food portions or levels of saturated fats in fast foods on obesity among particular cohorts at key points in life or for particular time periods.

The Social Change Model is also consistent with the Framework for Population Health – a widely accepted approach for organizing the social determinants of health that, in the early 1990s, was developed by the Canadian federal government in collaboration with academic researchers (Health Canada, 1994). The Framework for Population Health uses a broad definition of health, one that emphasizes building capacity for individuals and communities to maximize their health and well-being. It proposes an action strategy to achieve population health formed into a pyramid structure representing the interconnections among macro, meso, and micro processes that directly and indirectly influence health (Health Canada, 1994). The top of the pyramid represents the goal of attainable population health status and is the result of three dynamic factors. Moving from the base to the pinnacle of the pyramid are (1) foundations for action, (2) collective factors, and (3) individual factors (Health Canada, 1994). The first set of factors includes tools and supports (research, information, and public policy). The middle and bottom sections of the pyramid cover the social determinants of health, which are divided into collective factors (social and economic environment, physical environment, and health services) and individual factors (personal health practices, individual capacity, and coping skills). Stemming from this model, the 'social determinants of health' approach has focused heavily on the role of material (e.g., economic or financial) and social (e.g., minority status, social support) aspects of inequality in health. This is based largely on strong and extensive evidence that occupational status, income, and education are associated with patterns of health status and health utilization (for review, see Raphael, 2004). And, more recently, cultural determinants, such as ethnocultural norms and values and those related to living in different regions of the country, are deemed to influence health independently, as well as in conjunction with socio-economic factors. For example, the concept of multiple jeopardy connotes the simultaneous, interacting effect of minority status, socio-economic status, and other factors such as age and gender on health and well-being (Chappell and Havens, 1980; Penning, 1983). Although the study of a full set of determinants of health is beyond the scope of this book, individual lifestyle factors, socio-economic status, and regional and health utilization factors will comprise our main foci. These elements represent salient determinants of health drawn from the Framework for Population Health.

What Are Healthy Lifestyles and Why Should We Study Them?

There is no agreed upon definition or theory of lifestyle as it pertains to health. So, let us begin by defining what is meant by *healthy lifestyles* and then place this conceptualization within the context of the more widely known *lifestyle approach* found in the health literature. It is proposed that the ways in which people initiate and maintain healthy lifestyles is a lifelong process that is shaped by complex and dynamic systems interacting among physiological, psychological, and social domains. At the more general level of lifestyles per se, the World Health Organization maintains that lifestyles comprise 'a range of socially determined patterns of behaviour and interpretations of social situations, developed and used jointly by the group to cope with life' (WHO, 1996:118). In this sense, healthy lifestyles and the specific health behaviours comprising them (e.g., physical activity level, smoking, and eating habits) are part of a broader lifestyle that is constructed by a person's social network, social status, social expectations, and health beliefs. For instance, elements of the social environment, and its more recent conceptualization as social capital, have been shown to influence health (Lomas, 1998; Yen and Syme, 1999), in part through the development of healthy lifestyles.

Similarly, according to the classic work of Weber (1946:192), 'status groups are stratified according to the principles of their consumption of goods as represented by special styles of life.' Healthy lifestyles can be understood therefore as a manifestation of these broader lifestyles that are connected to the knowledge, beliefs, and values that individuals place on health, and which are socially created through stratification and social support systems. For example, persons who have higher education tend to place greater importance on adopting activities that have known health benefits. Conversely, health behaviours such as smoking, diet, and exercise can be used as core indicators of these healthy lifestyles, as well as predictors, or 'risk factors' of illness or disease. These risk factors are also sometimes called 'personal health practices' or 'harmful substance avoidance' because they sometimes cluster together (Harris and Guten, 1979). It is interesting, however, that some research has discovered that most health behaviours in fact are not highly correlated (Krick and Sobal, 1990; Sobal, Revicki, and DeForge, 1992). This is not surprising given that health behaviours are complex and connected to the social context in which they are embedded.

A separate but parallel perspective has been termed the 'materialist approach,' which emphasizes the centrality of opportunity structures in achieving health, often associated with purchasing power and one's relationship to the generation of wealth, or the means of production from a Marxian viewpoint (Lock and Wister, 1992). For instance, persons with more financial capital can join more sports clubs. At a social level, healthy lifestyles are likely some combination of the two – a Weberian lifestyle approach that is a reflection of health knowledge, beliefs, and social status, coupled with a Marxian materialist approach stressing the salience of economic resources that stratify populations in terms not only of wealth and social class, but also healthy lifestyles, healthy behaviours, and ultimately health status. This integrated perspective also allows for the inclusion of culture, often connected to ethnicity, which also stratifies individuals with regard to key values, norms, and beliefs that have been established as determinants of health status and health utilization. Adding a full multidisciplinary dimension to this conceptualization, healthy lifestyles also develop out of the web of interrelationships among genetic predisposition, physiology, and personality, as well as these social domains.

Thus, healthy lifestyles entail clusters of health behaviours that influence the health risk faced by individuals as the result of life chances and choices, and the social context in which these occur. For example, smoking, obesity, and a sedentary level of physical activity are reflective of an unhealthy lifestyle that significantly inflates the probability that an individual will die of heart disease. Yet, the mere fact of engaging in one health behaviour or preventative health practice does not necessarily mean that a person will engage in others. And while healthy lifestyles are often indicative of routine or habitual behavioural patterns, they may transform over an individual's life course, which makes it necessary to examine age-related trends at the population level. For example, it is well known that exercise levels decline as an individual ages. Furthermore, while research typically studies individual health behaviour, such as smoking, it is imperative to study a number of these simultaneously if we are to accurately assess population health. Healthy lifestyles and health behaviours therefore will be used interchangeably in this book, although it is understood that health behaviours are indicators of broader lifestyle patterns. In this sense, it should be kept in mind that these concepts represent more than just the propensity to exercise or maintain a healthy weight – that they are also part of dynamic systems working at individual, family, community, and social levels.

It should be noted as well that healthy lifestyles assume an influence not only on the health status of individuals, but also of populations. For example, it has been noted by several authors that changing lifestyles, possibly related to advancements in education and standard of living, have contributed to increases in life expectancy, improved functional mobility, and a decrease in rates of disability of successive cohorts of elderly people (Crimmins and Saito, 2001; Mirowsky and Ross, 1998; Robert and House, 1996). Shifts in education or income at the population level over time therefore would expose more people to their positive benefits for healthy lifestyles and health status. There is no doubt that medical advancements, such as heart bypass surgery and hip replacements, coupled with better public health during the '60s and onward, have also shaped this trend. Albeit, a healthy lifestyle remains a pivotal cornerstone of explanations concerning health and illness, in part because it is viewed as a mutable aspect of an individual that can be moulded in such a way as to reduce the need for health care services. While a lifestyle approach has been criticized for 'blaming the individual,' it is clear that health behaviours transcend individual choice, and must be understood within the social contexts in which they occur. This entails the influence of social structure and inequality, as well as human agency.

So how effective have our explanatory models been in accounting for variation in healthy lifestyles? Most researchers would agree that our ability to explain health behaviors at the individual level has been modest. Between 20% and 40% of the total variance is typically explained in lifestyle behaviours such as obesity, physical activity, smoking, drinking, nutrition, diet, and so on. Also, behavioral change – that is, movement into and out of healthy or unhealthy patterns of behaviour – is even more difficult to explain because the reasons for these changes are multifaceted. Furthermore, we have had only partial success with interventions aimed at improving health behaviours such as diet and weight loss, improving physical activity, and encouraging the reduction of smoking and other addictions. While many interventions have succeeded in altering the targeted behaviour among the treatment group during the period they are enrolled in a study using a relatively intensive intervention, the length of program effect – that is, the degree to which the change in behaviour has been sustained after a person is no longer in the program – has been considerably less successful. For example, many weight loss and smoking cessation programs enjoy relative success for a significant number of participants while they are in the program, but often participants return to pre-program levels once it ends. Moreover, most interventions have not filtered throughout enough segments of society to influence population health significantly (Gutman and Wister, 1994; Spence, Shephard, Craig, and McGannon, 2001). The exception, health promotion media campaigns (e.g., for smoking and exercise) have reached a wide audience, but have received mixed scientific support for having a powerful enough effect to influence individual behaviour.

In fact, the proportion of the population following minimum guidelines of basic healthy lifestyle practices is far from adequate from a population health perspective. For example, it is shocking that, depending on the definition used, between 40% and 50% of North Americans aged 65 and over are sedentary in their level of physical activity. Rates of engaging in exercise or leisure activity for the total adult population are not significantly better. Also, the rates of obesity are on the rise – 15% of Canadians and over 20% of Americans have body mass index (BMI) scores of 30 or more, which is clearly indicative of poor lifestyles that pose a significant health risk for these individuals. Thus, it is imperative that we study healthy lifestyles, since they are part of the causal fabric determining the health status of individuals and the population health of nations.

Have Healthy Lifestyles Really Improved over Time?

There is controversy as to whether and to what extent we have improved our lifestyle behaviors over the last several decades due to our public health and health promotion efforts. Mortality rates for ischemic heart disease and certain cancers have decreased, while other diseases have increased over that time period. Lifestyle factors are deemed to play a significant role in the etiology of these diseases. But the debate continues surrounding the degree to which lifestyles are becoming healthier over time and whether part of the decline in certain disease and mortality rates are connected to these patterns.

There has also been speculation as to whether baby boomers are faring as well as mid-life persons of the same age a generation ago (e.g., in the 1970s) in terms of lifestyles and health. In its report, 'Wake Up Call to Canadian Baby Boomers,' the Heart and Stroke Foundation of British Columbia and Yukon (1996) compared risk factors for heart disease and stroke among baby boomers in the 1990s compared to adults the same age in the 1970s. It found that baby boomers are doing better in terms of smoking and weight, but they have not raised their exercise levels compared to adults of the same age in the 1970s, and fewer have a healthy blood pressure and a healthy serum cholesterol level. For example, the percentage of adults in the 1990s who exercise regularly was reported at 35% compared to 38% of adults the same age in the 1970s. The comparative percentages for a healthy blood pressure were 75% and 84%, respectively, and a healthy serum cholesterol level was reported to be 55% and 86% for adults in the 1990s compared to the 1970s. Although these analyses are only preliminary, because they are limited in their comparisons of only two time periods (termed 'simple time-series analysis') and combine many age groups, they do suggest that baby boomers may be prone to some unhealthy lifestyles, and they emphasize the urgency for further research.

Have Rates of Chronic Illness Decreased over Time?

In his seminal work, Fries (1983) argued that, if adult life expectancy is relatively constant, and if the period between chronic infirmity and death can be postponed, then morbidity will be compressed into a shorter period of time. Research has been relatively consistent in its support of an increase in disability-free life expectancy in a number of countries, including Canada, the United States, and France (Crimmins and Saito, 2001; Manuel and Schultz, 2001; Robine, Mormiche, and Sermet, 1998). This implies that as people are living longer they are also free of disability for longer periods before death. As previously discussed, this may be, in part, the consequence of a more effective and/or efficient medical system rather than a reduction in the prevalence of chronic diseases – those illnesses that tend to be treatable but not curable. However, it is necessary to examine specific chronic illnesses, given that they do not necessarily follow the same patterns, and may change according to shifts in health behaviours and their consequence on health, such as the rise in obesity on diabetes rates.

Most people will face chronic illness some time in their life. Prevalence rates of chronic illness are especially high among older persons. For example, the elderly exhibit the following rates: 43% arthritis; 36% hypertension; 16% heart disease; 12% diabetes; 6% bronchitis/emphysema; and 6% asthma (Statistics Canada, 1999a). Yet, there is a perception that some lifestyles have improved among midlife persons (aged 45–64) as well as among older persons (65+), which has helped to lower the prevalence of chronic conditions over the last several decades – an improvement due to the efforts of the 'new public health.' Statistics Canada (1999b) has conducted simple time-series comparisons of the prevalence of the major chronic conditions between 1978/79 and 1998/99 (a period of 20 years), which paints a less than rosy picture. Among midlife Canadians, significant decreases have been documented between 1978/79 and 1998/99 in the prevalence rates for arthritis/rheumatism, hypertension, heart disease, and bronchitis/emphysema (Statistics Canada, 1999b). But, striking and statistically significant increases have occurred in prevalence rates for diabetes, asthma, and migraine headaches.

Turning to the 65 and over group, no positive trends were identified for any of the major chronic illnesses based on comparisons between 1978/79 and 1998/99, and, moreover, rates of diabetes and asthma have actually risen (Statistics Canada, 1999b). In an analysis of the linked data housed at the Manitoba Centre for Health Policy, Menec, Lix, MacWilliam and Soodeen (2003) found that between 1985–87 and 1997 99, Manitobans aged 65 and over experienced fewer myocardial infarctions, strokes, cancer, and hip fractures, but had a higher prevalence of diabetes, hypertension, and dementia. Thus, there appear to be opposite trends occurring depending on the type of illness under investigation and the age group studied. Furthermore, whether the statistically significant drop in the prevalence of arthritis/rheumatism, hypertension, heart disease, and bronchitis/emphysema shown to occur among persons aged 45 to 64 between the late 1970s and the late 1990s (Statistics Canada, 1999b) will be sustained into old age, or whether some of these conditions will only be delayed, is another unanswered question.

There are additional gaps in knowledge to be considered. Since the lowering of the prevalence of some chronic conditions may be due to pharmacological treatments for various chronic conditions (e.g., hypertension) or improved screening and early intervention (e.g., breast and prostate cancer, arthritis), it cannot be assumed that lifestyles influence health independent of other causal factors, including the primary care health system. Indeed, Evans et al. (2001) have shown that there has been substantive growth in the supply side of the formula that is within the health care industry, which has likely contributed to the escalation of utilization rates. Another issue is whether lifestyle change or an upturn in standard of living, or both, are influential in shaping these patterns. Population-level improvements in educational attainment, a rise in real income, and a more equitable distribution of income in society may all contribute to better health status.

The healthy lifestyle-chronic illness connection therefore implores further analyses. This is underscored by the enormous costs of chronic illness to the health care system. It is estimated that the total cost of cardiovascular disease (the most costly diagnostic category) on the health care sector in 1998 was $18.5 billion (11.6% of the costs of all illnesses), with a direct cost of $6.8 billion (8.1% of the total direct cost of all illnesses) (Health Canada, 1998a). Musculoskeletal diseases and cancer ranked second and third, accounting for $16.4 billion and $14.2 billion, respectively, in total costs; and $2.6 billion and $2.5 billion, respectively, in direct costs (Health Canada, 1998a). *Direct costs* pertain to hospitals, drugs, physicians, and institutions, while *indirect costs* include lost economic output due to disability and premature death. As people continue to live longer, and the population ages, there is no doubt that management of chronic illness will be a necessary prerequisite to a healthy population, and that patterns of lifestyle behaviours will be a major component to any formula for healthy aging.

Does Increased Immigration over Time Affect Population Health?

Consideration of changing patterns of population health also begs the question of whether the increasingly multicultural face of Canadian society has contributed to some of these health trends. It was noted earlier that immigration patterns affect the size of the baby boomer cohorts as they age. In addition, persons moving to Canada may not have experienced the same generational events, adding to the heterogeneity of what we call the baby boomers. Statistics Canada (1998a) has determined that 17.4% of the Canadian population is composed of persons who have been born outside of Canada, what we term immigrants. In 2001, about a quarter of a million (252,088) immigrants entered Canada (Statistics Canada, 2001a). This can be compared to 100,967 in 1978, which constitutes the beginning point of our trend analyses. The percentage increase between 1978 and 2001 is therefore a remarkable 150%. However, immigration numbers have been highly variable over the last several decades. For example, there were 84,518 in 1979; 143, 616 in 1980; 83,691 in 1985; 202,979 in 1990; 220,123 in 1995; and 205,711 in 2000.

Furthermore, the country of origin of immigrants has shifted dramatically over the last several decades, in part because of changing policies (see Boyd and Vickers, 2000, for review). For example, the proportion of all immigrants originating from the United Kingdom and Europe dropped from 90.3% prior to 1961, to about 19% between 1991 and 1996 (Statistics Canada, 1998a). Conversely, those stemming from Asian and Middle Eastern countries made up only 3% of all immigrants prior to 1961, compared to 57.1% between 1991 and 1996 (Statistics Canada, 1998a). It is also known that the bulk of immigrants are young or middle-aged adults, many of whom are now members of the baby boom age cohorts. This means that the health dynamics of baby boomers include not only movement of all birth cohorts along the age escalator, but also comparisons of Canadian-born and foreign-born individuals.

The steadily increasing importance of immigration in Canada has led to research into its implication for health status and health care utilization in recent years. Indeed, there has been a growing literature on this topic that has converged on two major patterns. First, it has been found that mortality and morbidity tend to be lower among immigrants than among the Canadian-born population, termed the *healthy immigrant effect*, and second, that the two groups begin to resemble one another with longer duration of residence in terms of health status indicators, even after controlling for the effects of age (Chen, Ng, and Wilkins, 1996; Chen, Wilkins and Ng, 1996; Federal, Provincial and Territorial Advisory Committee on Population Health, 1999). Relevant to this book, this converging pattern is observed for chronic illnesses, including arthritis, diabetes, and diseases of the circulatory system (Chen, Ng and Wilkins, 1996; Perez, 2002b; Rogers, 2003). However, the 'effect' is moderate, typically resulting in a relative risk, around 1.5 to 2. Thus, while the health of immigrants is better than average upon entry to this country, these differences are in the moderate range in terms of strength, and gradually disappear and become non-significant after about 10 years or so.

One explanation for the better health status of immigrants is a positive selection effect, whereby immigrants entering Canada tend to be better off financially, and those in poor health would be disallowed entry (Chen, Wilkins and Ng, 1996; Trovato, 1993). This is, in part, because of the application of immigration policy, but is also due to the socio-economic characteristics of immigrants. A second explanation is the cultural buffering hypothesis (Marmot, 1993), which contends that immigrants from less modern societies have more healthy lifestyles than the native-born population (e.g., diet, exercise, etc.) and strong norms that limit high-risk behaviours (e.g., lower propensity of heavy drinking).

Accounts of the gradual convergence in health status over time have been formed around two factors: socio-economic status (SES), and acculturation. Some researchers contend that the socio-economic disadvantages faced by immigrants are deleterious to their health and eventually disintegrates their initial health status advantage over the native-born population (Dunn and Dyck, 2000). However, most research indicates that the SES of foreign-born persons improves with longer duration of residence, which runs opposite to the above trend (Rogers, 2003). Moreover, education and income do not explain away the pattern of decreasing health status among immigrants with longer duration in the host country. Acculturation has also been used as an explanation for these patterns based on the notion that foreign-born individuals gradually conform to the cultural beliefs and practices of the host society. Thus, it might be argued that the decline in health status among immigrants is the result of their adopting the poorer lifestyle practices (diet, exercise, smoking, etc.) followed in Canadian society. Research by Rogers (2003) provides partial support for this notion; however, even after controlling for age, sex, SES, several health behaviours, and other determinants of chronic illness, the influence of duration of residence persists.

Furthermore, research has established that immigrants arrive in Canada in better health than the native-born population, but eventually lose their advantage, and resemble other Canadians in their health profile, even in midlife and later life (Gee, Kobayashi, and Prus, 2004). Since the majority of immigrants tend to be in their young adult or midlife years, and immigration has increased especially in the 1990s, there is little doubt that it has influenced population health. But it is also apparent that there may be a degree of cancelling out of some of these associations between immigration patterns and population health. We can state several conclusions: (1) the healthy immigrant effect is modest in its association with health status variables; (2) it wanes over time; and (3) it is likely not a significant factor associated with lifestyle changes. It does, however, warrant our attention when examining baby boomer health trends.

What Might the Future Health Status of Baby Boomers Look Like?

It is not uncommon to read contradictory reports about what Canada's health system will be like when baby boomers are in their golden years. Some researchers suggest that older baby boomers will be 'healthier and wealthier' than the current generation of elderly, and therefore will be less of a burden on the health care system (Blanchette and Valcour, 1998). Other reports paint a grimmer picture, suggesting that baby boomers will live longer, but in more years of chronic illness, and will expect and demand more health services that will not be available under the current system (Dychtwald, 1997). Media reports reflect these contradictory opinions, and will likely continue to do so because of the diversity of popular images that are espoused and embraced by individuals concerning the baby boomer generation. For example, some media articles report that baby boomers will break the social security bank when they draw pensions in large numbers, whereas others contend that baby boomers are the most financially secure and health conscious of all generations, with the opposite effect. The lack of empirical evidence has left conjecture and guesswork to dominate these debates.

There are, however, other major health trends that shed further light on this question. Research carried out on morbidity, life expectancy, and disability-free life expectancy indicates that as people live longer they are reporting more chronic illnesses, but with a decrease in long-term disability (Crimmins, 1996; Manton, Stallard, and Corder, 1997: Robine et al., 1998). This research has established that the seriousness of disability has declined over time, perhaps due to healthier lifestyles and the development of better treatment of illness. Concurrently, rates of dementia are expected to rise into the next century (Canadian Study of Health and Aging Working Group, 1994). It is estimated that approximately 8% of persons aged 65 and over, and 34.5% of persons aged 85 and over, have some form of dementia, and that rates have yet to reach a peak. Perhaps it is not surprising to observe that certain diseases will likely become more prevalent as the life expectancy of a nation rises, since most people must die from some epidemiological cause.

What we do not know is whether there is a general trend of improved health over time, or whether certain patterns are simply the result of expanded awareness of chronic illnesses and better diagnostics. Analyses of cohort patterns in health may help to answer these questions. Moreover, examination of age-related health trajectories without assessing age, period, and cohort effects in a population may result in serious misinterpretation of data. All too often, researchers assume linear trends in their predictions, typically by applying population projections to current age-specific rates, which lead to erroneous conclusions more often than not.

As evidenced in the study conducted by the Heart and Stroke Foundation of British Columbia and Yukon, with its alarmist title – 'Wake Up Call to Canadian Baby Boomers' – there is also a tendency for non-profit and non-governmental organizations to paint a rather bleak picture for the future. This may be, in part, related to more intensive competition over funding. It should be noted, however, that this particular study did not disaggregate the data into smaller cohorts (i.e., 5-year age-sex groups), only used two time points, and did not adequately address age, period, and cohort issues. Thus, their conclusions remain tenuous and unsubstantiated, albeit well publicized in the national media.

How Will Aging Baby Boomers Affect Health Care Utilization?

Probably the most important issue facing Canadians in the new millennium is the future of the Canadian health care system. Per capita spending on health care in Canada has risen steadily since the 1970s (with some small fluctuations in the 1990s), and it is recognized that the support of a publicly funded health care system may soon reach its limit. Central to this discussion is the role of population aging, typically defined as the increasing percentage of elderly in the population, on inflation of health care costs. Public perceptions have generally been negative – population aging will 'bankrupt' all publicly financed systems, including health care and the pension systems.

Research into the relationship between population aging and the utilization of health services has established that the aging of the population itself is not responsible for the rise in health care spending. An authoritative study has been conducted by Evans et al. (2001). Utilizing British Columbia's Linked Health Data Set, these researchers were able to combine several sources of administrative health data from the Medical Services Plan, Pharmacare, and hospital records. They estimate that between 1969 and 1985, only about 8% of the increase in hospital days in British Columbia over that 16-year period had been due to changes in the age structure (Evans et al., 2001). Age-specific changes in rates of hospital utilization, however, display dramatic shifts across the ages over the same period. Declines were experienced in all age groups except two: 75 to 84 (54.6% increase) and 85 and over (224.8% increase). These exceptional trends have been associated with a rise in the proportion of acute care days, because of more surgery (but with a decline in length of stay), and sharp inclines in extended care among the oldest age groups.

Turning to pharmaceuticals, total expenditures on drugs has more than tripled between 1985 and 1999, rising a remarkable 9% a year, compared to about 5.5% per year for hospitals and physicians' services (Evans et al., 2001). Part of the increase is attributed to the costs of stronger doses and more advanced chemical entity of drugs. But even the per capita ingredient costs of drugs, which accounts for the dosage, has ballooned 147% between 1985 and 1999 in BC, and this even covers the period when policy changes enforced the use of more generic versions of drugs. Evans et al. (2001) argue that approximately half of the augmentation in pharmaceutical costs has occurred for two therapeutic classes of drugs – hypertension drugs to control blood pressure, and antilipemic agents to control cholesterol levels. Both treatments respond to risk factors for cardiovascular disease. The authors contend that it has not been established that many of these higher-priced drugs (e.g., ACE inhibitors, and calcium channel blockers) are more effective than their cheaper predecessors. However, it should be noted, first, that the evidence on the efficacy of these drugs requires long-term analysis, and second, that there is evidence based on expert panel reviews for the use of ACE inhibitors and channel blockers under specific circumstances, and that the problem is the routine prescribing of these and other drugs by a subset of physicians (see CACR, 1999).

Population aging has been found to have an even smaller effect for utilization of doctor services. Barer et al. (1995) estimate that only 4.4% of the increase of physician fee-for-service payments (almost doubling between 1974/ 75 and 1985/86) is the result of shifts in the age structure. Higher physician payments for services have occurred among every age group, but, as expected, the rate is again highest for the oldest ones. For example, the growth in physician payments for 15- to 24-year-olds during this period is 25.1%, but for the 65 to 74 and 75 to 84 age groups, the rate of increase is 44.0% and 80.6%, respectively. Although physician supply rose 1.6% annually during this period (Barer et al. 1995), some researchers contend that rising educational attainment over recent decades, and therefore health knowledge, has made seniors more demanding of health services. This has been especially problematic during the recent expansion of health technology, such as the common use of MRIs and CAT scans for exploratory intervention and diagnoses. Black, Roos, Havens, and MacWilliam (1995) drew the same conclusion after finding that one half of the increase in specialist consultations by older Manitobans from 1971 to 1983 was due to more visits by people self-reporting themselves as in 'good health.' These research findings underline the need to conduct research into changing patterns, not only of health utilization, but also of health status and key determinants of health (e.g., lifestyle and socio-economic factors), and to juxtapose the two. Furthermore, once the baby boom generation moves into its senior years, especially into the 75 and over category, trends of significance may be greatly magnified because of the growing number of individuals experiencing these patterns (Carrière and Légaré, 1993). Thus, although population aging is not deemed to be the main culprit of steadily rising per capita health care costs, the sheer size of the baby boom generation will undoubtedly have a strong influence on resource allocation and policy development in all financial and health sectors. This will be most pronounced in the area of health care, our largest social expenditure ($110 billion annually), for which health status changes and health utilization patterns are in need of careful monitoring and examination. To this end, the heterogeneity of the baby boom generation in terms of determinants of health, health status, and health utilization, both across age-sex-specific cohorts and key socio-economic factors (such as education, income, employment status, etc.), has yet to be studied in enough detail to gain an informed understanding of their ramifications for the future of health care in Canada (Jenkins, Carrière and Légaré, 1997).

Advancements in Healthy Lifestyle Interventions

It is also insightful to consider developments in the area of lifestyle intervention research. Attempts to change health behaviours through programmatic interventions have been relatively successful in terms of demonstrating positive effects among persons while they remain in those programs. For example, persons of all ages and frailty levels exhibit significant improvement in outcomes during physical training interventions (see for example, Hickey, Wolf, Robins, and Harik, 1995; King, Rejeski, and Buchner, 1998; Spence et al., 2001). But, as we have seen, these interventions suffer from a major drawback – they often do not last. Smoking cessation and diet programs, for instance, have had high success rates while individuals are in the program, but do not fair as well when follow-ups are conducted after a significant period of time, due to the propensity for people to relapse. Moreover, effect sizes of these interventions (i.e., the program impact on people's behaviour) tend to be modest, mainly because of limited intensity, duration, frequency, and content of such interventions, and because behaviour change is difficult.

It is also common for programs to attract participants who often benefit the least – those in better health, and persons who have stronger social support systems and higher socio-economic statuses. These tend to be the same individuals who are motivated to make lifestyle gains, so that we are often 'preaching to the converted.' Similarly, there is a tendency for many programs to lose participants for whom they would provide benefit due to attrition from the start of the program until its completion (Prohaska, 1998). For these reasons, dissemination and diffusion of intervention knowledge and practice to communities and the larger society has been slow (see International Longevity Centre, 2000). At this point, we should not expect lifestyle interventions to 'fix' lifestyle problems identified among the baby boomers.

Yet, we have observed a number of notable advancements in recent years in the field of prevention research. The number and quality of randomized clinical trial evaluation studies have reached a critical mass in many health fields (e.g., cardiovascular and diabetes prevention), which has allowed for meta-analyses and expert panel reviews of these studies (CACR, 1999; Wing, Goldstein, Acton, Birch, Jakicic, Sallis, Smith-West, Jeffery, and Surwit, 2001). These approaches assess the quality of research and identify replication of results of those studies that meet a designated level of scientific rigor. To some extent, we are now able to identify what works for whom, for how long, and why. Unfortunately, most of this work pertains to a specific disease, rather than to primary prevention. Other promising findings have also emerged from intervention programs, such as the benefits enjoyed by individuals who volunteer (especially as leaders of programs), programs that target specific groups in society (frail elderly), and community empowerment approaches in lieu of individual-based interventions (Ory and DeFriese, 1998). Furthermore, innovations in the area of lifestyle health promotion that can be implemented in partnership with the primary care system, with the support and involvement of physicians (e.g., especially smoking cessation and exercise programs), also appear to be effective (Prohaska, 1998). For example, two exercise counselling programs, differing in the number of contacts with primary care practitioners, raised cardiovascular fitness (i.e., lung capacity measured as Vo2 max) for women compared to recommended care (Writing Group for the Activity Counseling Trial Research Group, 2001). Given that the majority of health care resources are used in acute care, primary care, and rehabilitative services, efforts to enhance lifestyle health behaviours through the health care sector have not received much attention beyond fragmented efforts at smoking cessation and weight control.

Finally, interventions using Web-based approaches to lifestyle change have been on the rise, given that approximately 70% of households in urban areas have Internet access. Most of these efforts tend to provide only health information, without the strong motivational components necessary to alter behaviour in an effective and sustained manner. Two well-known ones are the Canadian Health Network and WebMD. However, the more sophisticated Internet programs that have been developed recently tend to target risk behaviours among persons with a known disease, such as the D-Net diabetes self-management program (McKay, King, Eakin, Seeley, and Glasgow, 2001; Glasgow, Boles, McKay, Feil, and Barrera, 2003). D-Net includes goal-setting, personalized feedback, strategies to overcome barriers to exercise, availability of an email 'personal coach' and a peer support chat area. Moreover, there is little doubt that we can anticipate further development of Web-based health promotion programs with the spread of information technology. One of these is in the area of smoking cessation programming (Lenert, Munoz, Stoddard, Delucchi, Bansod, Skoczen, and Perez-Stable, 2003), but others will likely include physical activity, diet, and weight control, and will target cardiovascular disease and other chronic conditions. Although Internet approaches to health promotion have the potential to reach broad segments of the population at relatively low expense, the research to date is in its infancy and has not yet firmly established its efficacy and effectiveness.

Overall, advancements and innovations in prevention research in all probability will play a decisive role in determining healthy lifestyles and population health in the decades to come. However, their success will depend not only on research and policy developments, but also on the theories underlying them.

3

Advancements in Healthy Lifestyle Theories: Towards Transdisciplinarity

Understanding Healthy Lifestyles

How are healthy lifestyles developed, sustained, and changed as we age? There are a number of theoretical approaches that have either directly or indirectly addressed this question. The current stage of development in theoretical knowledge is one in which synthesis of ideas, often from multidisciplinary fields with differing foci, is occurring. As previously discussed in Chapter 2, the Social Change Model integrates elements of age stratification, life course, and cohort approaches to the study of health behaviour. This model is dynamic in its recognition of interlocking spheres of individual and structural factors that manifest themselves in changing cohort experiences and ultimately population health. The Framework for Population Health, also introduced in the last chapter, is a common template for modelling what are known as the determinants of health.

While the above-mentioned approaches provide a foundation for our understanding of the nexus of healthy lifestyles and population health, there are a number of additional theories that have also generated considerable research and knowledge. A brief review of these is required in order to elaborate how lifestyle behaviours unfold over the course of people's lives. Found in the fields of gerontology, demography, sociology, psychology, public health, epidemiology, and human ecology, these multidisciplinary approaches provide the contextual and theoretical depth underlying social change and population health. While not meant to be exhaustive, advancements in the following four perspectives and theories epitomize the movement towards greater transdisciplinarity across micro-meso-macro-level domains. These perspectives and theories are consistent with our conceptualization of healthy lifestyles, and provide greater depth and detail to the Social Change Model and the Framework for Population Health. It will be observed that, while each makes a unique contribution to the puzzle of healthy lifestyles, they also share a number of assumptions with the Social Change Model.

The Developmental Perspective

The developmental perspective, as applied to health, focuses on the combination of psychosocial (self-efficacy or confidence) and material influences (socio-economic resources) in conjunction with biological factors that vary over the life course. Biological embedding is the process by which human experience influences the healthfulness of people as they age at the physiological level (Hertzman, 1998). Various types of resources (capital) are deemed to influence this process. For example, education is a form of human capital that assists in problem-solving skills and self-efficacy, and thus shapes healthy lifestyles throughout life (Mirowsky and Ross, 1998). Material resources (i.e., financial capital, distribution of wealth, etc.) play an obvious role in affecting life chances and conditions that may also determine short-term and long-term health. Additionally, there are a host of factors considered to be indicators of social capital (supportive networks), such as family stability, good schooling, community support, and positive peer interaction, which also have been found to generate good health outcomes later in life.

There is controversy in this literature, however, as to the importance of the timing of biological embedding for healthy lifestyle enhancement. This is reflected in what are known as the Latency and Pathways Models found in the developmental literature pertaining to health (Hertzman, 1998). On the one hand, the Latency Model suggests that there is a critical period in childhood development at which time certain attributes and skills need to be fostered for an individual to experience positive personal growth. On the other hand, the Pathway Model states that developmental deficiencies and instability in childhood, chronic stress, and physiological factors contribute to a cycle of social problems for some individuals, but that these may be overcome at later points in the life cycle. Examining results from relevant studies, especially the famous U.S. Perry Preschool Longitudinal Study, Hertzman argues that there is evidence supporting both models, and that this points to the need for intervention at various points over the life course of individuals and cohorts. Thus, the developmental perspective draws our attention to the principal conclusion that health promotion and population health initiatives can be effective when targeting people at any age, but that there may be particular junctures at which point people are most malleable.

There is also recognition of cascading effects over time, such that earlier health experiences may influence later ones in powerful ways. For instance, negative residential school experiences have been shown to have long-term consequences for the health and well-being of some First Nations individuals (Day, 2001). Additionally, activity patterns of older adults, for instance, are correlated with exercise history during midlife (Lalive d'Epinay and Bickel, 2003). Of course, special attention needs to be invested in children and youth, since many health and lifestyle skills, and patterns of behaviour, are moulded during the formative years and have long-term consequences. The assumptions rooted in the developmental perspective are analogous to the life course approach, which is also at the core of the Social Change Model.

The Social Capital Perspective

Social capital is defined as 'features of social organization such as networks, norms and trust that facilitate coordination and cooperation for mutual benefit' (Lomas, 1998:1183). This approach points to the social forces located within the family, social networks, and community, rather than merely those associated with the individual, that may influence health. Positive normative milieus embedded within strong social links are viewed as non-monetary resources that may facilitate an individual, family, or community to maximize human potential (Coleman, 1988). Research has demonstrated the efficacy of community development approaches as well as many aspects of the social network that can elevate health. For example, a persistent association has been found between social networks, social support, and health status (Berkman and Syme, 1979; Berkman, 1984; Chappell, 1992); the impact of neighbourhood and housing environments on health (Dunn and Hayes, 2000; Wister, in press); and the beneficial influence of mutual aid and self-help group participation on illness management through self-care (Gottlieb, 2000; Wister, 1995). Empowering and developing capacity at the community level for primary prevention of disease through lifestyle enhancement may prove to be as important as individual-level programs. In addition, family-based approaches to certain lifestyle behaviours, such as nutrition and weight control, may be shown in time to be at least as effective as targeting individuals, given that families share many foods and eating habits. It is also noteworthy that social capital, although distinguished from financial capital, has been found to be associated with socio-economic status. It appears that persons with material advantages tend to be able to access stronger levels of social capital throughout life. Thus, there are some interactional effects among these types of capital that may magnify their impact on immediate, short-term, and long-term health outcomes.

Furthermore, underlying the concept of social capital is an enormous literature that has demonstrated the role that social support plays in one's health (for review, see Chappell, 1992). Social support has been conceptualized more broadly than social capital, including both emotional and instrumental types of support stemming from myriad connecting points of the support network (family, friends, services, etc.). This research has established that social support can have a direct positive influence on health as well as a buffering effect, the latter of which can limit the negative consequences of life stressors on health outcomes. Some of the benefits of social support include perceptions of affective support; for instance, the belief that the individual has significant others in their life to whom they can turn when in need. Other benefits entail the day-to-day provision of emotional and instrumental support that may alleviate stress and meet a variety of personal needs.

Kahn and Antonucci (1980) have introduced the notion of *convoys of support*, representing the fluidity of the support network that may follow an individual as he or she ages, and which is also consistent with a life course perspective. While it is understood that social support systems change shape dramatically as one moves through various life stages, there can also be a degree of continuity of support invested in the individual over many years in the form of relationship bonds. For instance, research has shown that marital history can be an important determinant of formal support use in later life (Wister and Dykstra, 2000). Thus, by merging the concepts of social support and social capital, it is clear that there are components of the social fabric of society that have far-reaching consequences for our health. These elements need to be recognized in our understanding of health behaviours and status, as well as of health promotion strategies.

The Transtheoretical Model and Stage Theories

A major development in the explication of healthy lifestyles in recent years has occurred in the domain of behavioural change theories (for discussion, see especially Weinstein, Rothman and Sutton, 1998). These micro, or individual, approaches have shifted attention from analyses of health behaviours at a particular point in time to studying what moves people through intention-behaviour transitions. The Transtheoretical Model (TM) is one of a family of social-psychological behavioural change models that was originally formulated to understand smoking cessation and other addictive behaviours (Prochaska, DiClemente, and Norcross, 1992). Since that time, it has been applied to many other lifestyle behaviours, in particular, exercise (e.g., Marcus and Owen, 1992; Courneya, 1995). The TM assumes that individuals spiral through five progressive stages of change, from thinking about changing behaviour to actually making the behaviour a habit: precontemplation, contemplation, preparation, action, and maintenance. *Precontemplation* occurs when a person has no intention of altering his or her present health behaviour, such as exercising. *Contemplation* transpires when a person is considering a change in the health behaviour, but does not intend to do so over the next six months. *Preparation* is present when an individual makes a behavioural change but has not adopted the behaviour completely. *Action* occurs when a person has engaged in the behaviour, such as regular exercise, for less than six months. Finally, the *maintenance* stage is when a person has sustained the behaviour for a period longer than six months (Prochaska, DiClemente, and Norcross, 1992). Although there remains some controversy around the extent to which persons spiral up and down the stages in a sequential manner, especially when managing a chronic illness (Wister and Romeder, 2002), there is ample evidence demonstrating that the stage of behavioural change at which people find themselves begs a specific type of health promotion approach. It also raises issues of individual motivation and other major decision-making components.

Social learning concepts such as *self-efficacy* (perceived confidence in ability to control behaviour), and those drawn from the Theory of Planned Behaviour (TOPB) – involving intentions, attitudes, norms, and control – also have been incorporated into this approach to help explain why individuals move from one stage to another (Fishbein and Ajzen, 1975; Godin, 1994). These concepts have also been applied specifically to the understanding of self-care practices among older persons managing a chronic illness (Clark, 1996; McDonald-Miszczak, Wister, and Gutman, 2001). Seminal work by Bandura (1977) and his colleagues has established that self-efficacy evaluations influence choice, effort expenditure, thoughts, emotional reactions, and behavioural performance (Clark, 1996; Marcus, Selby, Niaura, and Rossi, 1992). In other words, individuals must believe that they have the skills necessary to engage in particular health behaviour, such as exercise, in order to successfully perform it. Research tends to show that it is important to make a behavioural change appear attainable and enjoyable to enhance alterations in lifestyle behaviours (Clark, 1996).

The Theory of Planned Behavior emphasizes normative factors, such as expectations of health behaviour and its perceived importance for an individual, as well the importance of triggering an intention to change (Godin, 1994). It also parallels the well-known Health Belief Model (HBM), which stresses the weighing of costs and benefits associated with health decisions based on belief structures (Rosenstock, 1974). There has been mounting evidence in support of these social-psychological dimensions. For example, research into factors that predict exercise stage has identified that intention to change, knowledge, and importance of its benefits, as well as family support of exercise, are central to change processes (Lee, 1993; Marcus et al., 1992; Marcus, Bock, and Pinto, 1997). Thus, visualizing lifestyle changes as important for one's health, and the power of expectations or norms surrounding these behavioural shifts, are fundamental components of health promotion and population health.

The strength of the synthesis of these social-psychological-stage models is that they emphasize the salience of tailoring health promotion efforts depending on an individual's readiness to improve behaviour, in tandem with a number of salient objective and subjective attributes of the individual. The decision-making process underlying stage movement is obviously complex. The normative environment is a powerful force that affects expectations surrounding behaviour. Self-efficacy, or confidence, is a necessary precursor to making a shift in behaviour. And intentions to change and cues to initiate a successful transition are important prerequisites. At the heart of social-psychological models of health behaviour is motivation. This being the case, media campaigns, for example, need to foster clear and attainable healthy prescriptions of healthy behaviour (and proscriptions for unhealthy ones); emphasize the importance of health, and the seriousness and consequences of unhealthy behaviour; facilitate a greater sense of confidence in being able to make a change, and enjoyment in its attainment; and contain tailored messages and cues for individuals at different stages of readiness. The provision of health information without these crucial elements is likely to produce little in the way of population health. However, the social-psychological theories are limited by their focus on the individual. Thus, other approaches have developed that link the individual and structural processes underlying health behaviour and health status, to which we now turn.

The Social Ecology of Health Promotion

A Social Ecological Model of health promotion has been developed that is probably the most multidisciplinary framework addressing pathways to health (McMichael, 1999). A noteworthy example is Stokols (1992), who integrates interdisciplinary research literature into a systems model drawing on the seminal work of Antonovsky (1979). The fundamental assumptions are that (1) healthfulness is the result of a complex interplay of facets of the physical environment, social environment, and personal factors, including genetic heritage, psychological predispositions, and behavioural patterns; (2) environments can be described along several dimensions, including subjective-objective levels, proximate-distal ones, and independent (e.g., space and pollution), or composite factors (e.g., behavioural and social contexts) with an emphasis on positive environmental resources; and (3) participants within these environmental contexts can be studied as interlocking systems at individual, group, family, community, or population levels (Stokols, 1992:7–8). Recent developments of this model make use of it to translate theory to practice in health promotion (Best, Stokols, Green, Leischow, Holmes, and Buchholz, 2003).

From this perspective, healthy lifestyles can be understood within a number of overlapping spheres covering the full micro-meso-macro continuum – that is, individual, programmatic, and social-structural domains. Added to this, it emphasizes the centrality of the physical milieu stemming from the person-environment paradigm (Wister, in press). The physical and social environments can function as mediums for health (e.g., nutrients in food) or disease transmission (e.g., fatty acid content in food). They can also operate as a stress reducer, or stressor (e.g., flexibility in work or changing work demands). As a source of support, safety, or danger, the physical and social milieu can retard or exacerbate disablement, and may directly influence the risk of morbidity or mortality (such as through the absence of safe biking and walking paths to facilitate exercise and reduce the risk of accidents). They can also enable or act as a barrier for health behaviour (e.g., accessibility of health care), and provide health resources (e.g., well-organized community health promotion). The interaction of personal and environmental factors situated within a social-ecological systems model can therefore influence health trajectories both directly and indirectly, through a myriad of channels, and may do so through both salutogenic (positive) and pathogenic (negative) pathways (Wister, in press). Some of the most powerful evidence supporting this model stems from health-policy analysis. For example, research has shown that there are intended and unintended consequences of raising tobacco taxes, thereby raising the cost of cigarettes. On the one hand, this may reduce smoking because of the cost constraint, and generate financial support for the health care system. On the other hand, it can result in an increase in smuggling and underground markets. This reinforces the need to carefully examine health policy at different levels of analysis and across these various domains.

Emerging Transdisciplinary Paradigms: The Chinese Boxes

Based on these and other theories, a number of epidemiologists and social ecologists argue for the development of a new paradigm in response to the recent era of theoretical pluralism termed *eco-epidemiology* (McMichael, 1999; Susser and Susser, 1996a, 1996b). As a starting point, they propose a paradigm that links nested and interlocking layers of causal factors, termed the *Chinese Boxes*. The associated analytical approach identifies determinants and outcomes at different levels of organization: within and between contexts (using new information systems), and in depth (using new biological systems) (Susser and Susser, 1996a, 1996b). One dimension of this framework is the inherent connectedness among domains, such as populations, communities, single individuals, and individual biological systems. A second dimension is the importance of specifying and elaborating the underlying causal processes affecting health and illness. Applied herein, these are deemed to be essential in order to understand how healthy lifestyles influence population health, and how they can be enhanced through various types of interventions. Furthermore, the conceptualization of health as a series of Chinese Boxes entices us to continually dig deeper into the etiology and causal fabric of health and illness. The social-ecological approach and the Chinese Boxes paradigm certainly share many facets with respect to multiple spheres of influence, also inherent in the Social Change Model. Most important, however, is that these models emphasize the need for transdisciplinary progression. The study of healthy lifestyles and population health provides us with an ideal context.

Beyond the Human Genome Project: Lifestyle Pathways Are Also Important

In recent years, we have observed considerable interest in the Human Genome Project, and similar projects in which scientists are attempting to identify genes within the DNA structure that can be linked causally to diseases. Led by Francis Collins, the U.S. Human Genome Project began in 1990 coordinated by the Department of Energy and the National Institutes of Health. Another, private endeavour led by Craig Venter of Celera Genomics, has worked in parallel with the publicly funded project and both have reported on the sequencing of the human genome. Other research groups have been established throughout the world targeting specific groupings of genes. They report approximately 30,000 genes and three billion chemical base pairs that comprise the human DNA (Human Genome Project Information, 2003). Expectations have continued to build about the potential benefits of this research for the health of individuals and populations, in particular its use in pinpointing the genetic causes of health and disease and the pursuit of cures.

While this research is extremely valuable and we have yet to fully appreciate and realize its potential, there are good reasons to continue study into lifestyle and environmental causes of disease. Alterations in health and illness are extremely variable over time and place, thus making genetic explanations incomplete. Furthermore, the research evidence suggests that lifestyles explain at least as much variation in health and illness as do genes. One piece of evidence is the fact that the doubling of the prevalence of diabetes in Canada and the United States over the last two decades cannot be attributed solely to genetic predisposition, since modifications or mutations in our genetic makeup occur over multiple generations, not decades. Also, although family history of disease is a definite predisposing factor for a number of chronic illnesses, research suggests that the interaction of family history and lifestyle add an important dimension to the understanding of the etiology of disease. For example, a study by Chen and Millar (2001a) has shown that physical activity level has a protective effect for the incidence of cardiovascular disease even among persons with a family history of heart disease. Thus, a stronger explanatory framework would emphasize the interaction among lifestyle behaviours, exposure to environmental elements, and genetic factors, and will definitely provide the best solutions and treatment options in the long term.

It is also important to recognize that there may be both positive and negative pathways by which lifestyles influence health. In his seminal work, Antonovsky (1979) introduced the term *salutogenesis* to refer to the understanding of the etiology of emotional and physical well-being that may contribute directly or indirectly to disease or illness. Exercise is an example of a salutogenic pathway to health status because it may positively affect not only the physical components of health status, but also subjective ones, such as well-being, depression, and self-efficacy. There also may be pathogenic pathways to health that have a deleterious influence on health status, as evidenced by smoking or obesity; and, furthermore, the root causes of these unhealthy lifestyle behaviours. The principal idea is that we must move beyond proximate causes of health status and examine factors involved in the full developmental sequence of health and illness (McMichael 1999; Wister, 2004), and we must ultimately connect these to genetic predisposition. Investigation into healthy and unhealthy lifestyles is vital to elucidate the complex chain of causation underlying individual and population health. We turn now to four major lifestyle behaviours deemed to influence our health – smoking, physical activity, body mass/weight, and alcohol consumption – factors that comprise the focus of research in this book.

4

Linking Lifestyle Behaviours and Health

Smoking and Health

Evidence has been accumulating for the last 50 years that smoking tobacco products have serious deleterious health effects. In the mid-1960s, the U.S. surgeon general's office began to make unqualified announcements concerning the harmful effects of tobacco (U.S. Department of Health and Human Services, 2000). Parallel developments were occurring in Canada at approximately the same time. According to the 2000/01 Canadian Community Health Survey (CCHS), approximately 22% of Canadians aged 15 and over smoke regularly, down almost one-half from about 40% in the late 1970s. However, while smoking prevalence rates have decreased in both the United States and Canada since that time, they are still considered to be high, and smoking among young adults, especially young women, has actually been on the rise. Additionally, if we combine past and present smokers, the proportion of persons exposed to the detrimental effects of cigarettes is even more profound. From a global perspective, Canada is a good news–bad news nation. Of 87 countries examined by the World Health Organization in the mid-1990s, we ranked 72nd in smoking prevalence among males, but 7th for females (WHO, 1997). The high (negative) ranking for women is largely due to the fact that female smoking rates are relatively low in less developed countries thus far. Overall, we rank 13th in the world in the consumption of cigarettes. Thus, smoking remains a major social problem in Canada, one about which we should not become complacent.

Approximately 45,000 people died in Canada in 2002 because of smoking or environmental tobacco smoke (Health Canada, 2002). And one in five deaths are estimated to be smoking-related, contributing to the loss of five million years of potential lifespan of North Americans (U.S. Department of

Health and Human Services, 2000). It is therefore not surprising that smoking is considered to be the most influential lifestyle affecting people's health, one that contributes substantially to health care expenditures. Some estimates indicate that the direct and indirect costs of smoking in Canada range between $7.8 and $11.1 billion annually (Single, Robson, Xie, and Rehm, 1998), which approximate the total amount of tax revenues accrued from that source. What is problematic, however, is that many individuals begin to smoke and continue to smoke in the face of the insurmountable evidence pointing to its dangerous effects.

Indeed, there is an enormous body of literature that confirms relationships between smoking and a variety of health outcomes, including mortality (e.g., American Council on Science and Health, 1999; Lamarche, 1988; U.S. Department of Health, Education and Welfare, 1979; WHO, 1997). The most commonly cited harmful outcomes of smoking are for lung and respiratory disease, cancer, and cardiovascular disease. For example, smoking is the principal, preventable cause of cardiovascular disease; it increases mortality by 50% and doubles the incidence of cardiovascular disease (CACR, 1999; Ockene and Miller, 1997). However, smoking has been documented as a risk factor for many other chronic conditions, such as bronchitis, emphysema, digestive diseases, and musculoskeletal health, to name a few. Research also supports the negative effect of second-hand smoke on a host of chronic conditions, such as asthma, ischemic heart disease, and lung cancer (American Council on Science and Health, 1999; CDC, 2000; Wister and Gee, 1994).

Turning briefly to the determinants of smoking, there is strong evidence that there are a large number of physiological, psychological, and social factors that influence smoking. Smoking is highly addictive at both physiological and psychological levels, and it is affected by the cost and availability of cigarettes as well as by numerous social elements, such as peer group influence. In terms of age patterns, rates of smoking tend to peak in early adulthood and fall from midlife into the elder years. Furthermore, while the prevalence of smoking has declined over the last few decades, the smallest decrease has occurred among persons with lower education (high school or less) and income, especially women with these characteristics (Millar, 1996). Smokers with low education tend to be less influenced by media anti-smoking programs and report facing fewer smoking restrictions in their daily activities than do smokers with higher education (p. 11). Smoking also tends to be more prevalent among certain groups of immigrants; and there are regional variations, such as Quebecers exhibiting a greater propensity to smoke than persons from other provinces. Thus, smoking varies across several social dimensions, reflecting its multifarious nature and the diverse causal web surrounding it.

Lowering rates of smoking in the population is undoubtedly one of the most worthwhile health promotion initiatives in terms of potential health benefit, since it eliminates a major risk factor for a multitude of preventable diseases, as well as early death. While there has been progress in this regard, a significant proportion of the population continues to smoke. Additional research is needed to further detail smoking trends in order to make accurate predictions, and to pinpoint where our health promotion efforts should be concentrated. This is particularly challenging, given that many of the remaining smokers who have not been able to maintain a non-smoking stage – the 'diehard smokers' – are the most difficult to influence.

Physical Activity and Health

Persistent and confirmatory evidence has accumulated that maintaining adequate levels of physical activity and exercise also help individuals to prolong health and preserve a higher quality of life, especially as they age. However, even though most people are aware of the many benefits of physical activity, the proportion of the population that does not meet minimum recommended guidelines is extremely high in both Canada and the U.S. Spence et al. (2001) note that, while 81% of Canadians view physical activity as health enhancing, the majority (60%) report levels that are below those recommended by the *Canadian Physical Activity Guide to Healthy Active Living* (Health Canada, 1998b), a report providing specific activity levels. In addition, it is estimated that only 20% of Canadians are cognizant of these guidelines (Spence et al., 2001). More specifically, using the 1994/95 and 1998/99 National Population Health (NPH) surveys, Chen and Millar (1999) have estimated that a striking 40% of the Canadian adult population (aged 20 and over) do *not* engage in a level of physical activity considered to be at the extreme low end of an active lifestyle: brisk walking, running, aerobics, weight-bearing exercises, tennis, and so on, for at least 15 to 20 minutes in duration three or more times per week. Another 15% exercise at light-intensity regular levels; 22% exercise at moderate-intensity regular levels, and only 18% exercise at high-intensity levels on a regular basis. Furthermore, it is estimated that 64% of Canadian adults over the age of 18 exercise at levels that are insufficient for optimal health benefits (Spence et al., 2001).

Exercise patterns in the U.S. also do not appear to be healthy. Sherwood and Jeffery (2000) report that a shocking 78% of U.S. adults are not meeting the more strict levels of regular physical activity defined by the American College of Sports Medicine and the Centers for Disease Control: a minimum of 30 minutes of moderate to vigorous activity on most days of the week. And about

27% of American adults report that they never engage in physical activity during their leisure time (CDC, 2002). Rates of sedentary behaviour in Canada are only slightly lower. It also should be noted that individuals tend to overestimate self-reported physical activity and exercise patterns, which makes this an even more pressing social issue.

There are also contradictory reports pertaining to shifts in activity trends over the last several decades. Some published reports suggest that rates of physical activity peaked in the late 1980s and have subsequently decreased (see Health Canada, 1995). Others contend that inactivity levels declined between 1981 and the mid-1990s, but that 'progress has now stalled' (Spence et al., 2001:10). A more careful examination of recent trends is required that accounts for age-specific changes and which uses multiple surveys that better reflect changes that occur over that period. Regardless of the pattern over time, it is apparent that inactive lifestyles have become the norm for a large segment of our society. This high level of inactivity apparent in Canada today demands immediate attention among researchers, policy-makers, and practitioners.

The evidence for beneficial effects of physical activity continues to mount. There is a plethora of research that has established the health benefits of physical activity for mortality, morbidity, and quality of life across the life span (e.g., Chen and Millar, 1999; Health and Welfare Canada, 1988; Paffenbarger, Hyde, and Wing, 1990; Shepard and Montelpare, 1988). Furthermore, physical activity has been shown to play a role in both prevention and rehabilitation (McPherson, 1992). For example, exercise appears to have a beneficial impact for osteoporosis in women (Oyster, Morton, and Linnell, 1984), cardiovascular diseases (Haapanen, Miilunpalo, Vuori, Oja and Pasanen, 1997; Paffenbarger et al., 1990; Sesso, Paffenbarger, and Lee, 2000; Sesso, Paffenbarger, Ha, and Lee, 1999), diabetes (Haapanen et al., 1997), muscular strength, flexibility, and functional capacity (DiPietro, 2001; Frontera and Meredith, 1989; Spirduso and Gilliam-MacRae, 1991), the prevention of falls (Shepard, 1987), chronic pain management, such as for arthritis (Clark, Becker, Janz, Lorig, Rakowski and Anderson, 1991; Young, 1986), and longevity (Paffenbarger et al., 1990; Rakowski, 1992).

One authoritative study calculated the relative risk for various chronic diseases in Canada for levels of physical activity (Katzmarzyk, Gledhill, and Shephard, 2000). These researchers report that physically inactive Canadians are approximately 90% more likely to develop coronary artery disease; 60% more likely to suffer from osteoporosis; and 40% more likely to experience stroke, hypertension, colon cancer, or Type 2 diabetes. Furthermore, about one-third of coronary artery disease; one-quarter of osteoporosis; and one-fifth of stroke, hypertension, colon cancer, and Type 2 diabetes are the result of inactivity. In another notable study, Haapanen et al. (1997) followed a cohort of 1,340 men and 1,500 women aged 35 to 63 for a 10-year period in the U.S. and found that the relative risks after adjusting for age and smoking were 1.98 for CHD (coronary heart disease) incidence, 1.73 for hypertension, and 2.64 for diabetes, when comparing the lowest and highest three activity groups. Additionally, an American Heart Association expert panel review found conclusive evidence for the positive effect of exercise and physical activity for atherosclerotic cardiovascular disease (Thompson, Buchner, Pina, Balady, Williams et al., 2003). There are also numerous mental health benefits of physical activity and exercise. For example, these have been shown to prevent depression (Chen and Millar, 1999) and promote psychological well-being among persons at all points in the life cycle (Gauvin, Spence, and Anderson, 1999; Shepard, 1987).

Similar to smoking, the economic costs of physical inactivity are considerable. Katzmarzyk, Gledhill and Shephard (2000) have estimated that approximately 10% of all deaths are attributable to inactivity. They also estimate that about 25% of the health care costs (hospital care, medical care, drugs, and research) associated with treating coronary artery disease, stroke, colon cancer, breast cancer, Type 2 diabetes, and osteoporosis are directly related to inactivity. Thus, as a nation, there are many financial benefits that can be realized if we are able to significantly reduce the level of inactivity in Canada.

Attempts to manipulate activity levels through programs and efficacy interventions have met with considerable success based on a multitude of published evaluation studies (see Dishman and Buckworth, 1996; Dunn, Anderson, and Jakicic, 1998; King et al., 1998; and Spence et al., 2001, for reviews). However, effectiveness of interventions, such as community-based or school programs, have yet to receive the same level of supporting evidence. In fact, Spence, Shephard, Craig, and McGannon (2001) contend that based on accepted definitions of effectiveness, there is little or no scientific proof of successful community-based programs conducted in Canada.

So, what is it that is keeping us from developing and sustaining active lifestyles and healthy levels of strength training and aerobic exercise? There is an enormous literature that addresses the causal mechanisms underlying physical activity patterns. While a full discussion of these factors is beyond the scope of this book, it is valuable to touch briefly on the principal ones. As stated in a recent review by Sherwood and Jeffery (2000), physical activity is a complex, dynamic process that is influenced by a large number of rather diverse factors. The major determinants of exercise can be divided into two main groupings: individual characteristics and environmental characteristics. Individual factors pertain to psychosocial elements such as motivations, self-efficacy, exercise history, and other health beliefs and behaviours (Godin, 1994). It also includes attributes such as the age, gender, and socio-economic status (SES) of the individual. Environmental factors encompass such things as cost constraints, access, and time barriers, as well as social and cultural stresses and supports, and social change (Sherwood and Jeffery, 2000). Research shows that physical activity patterns are higher among younger and higher SES individuals with more active social networks, and among those who have higher exercise efficacy (confidence), and those who place greater importance on exercise. These persons also tend to have fewer material and psychological barriers to exercise, and maintain health beliefs that are consistent with that lifestyle. At the broader level, it has been argued by some researchers that the propensity for individuals to spend more time in front of computers and televisions, longer times in cars, and ultimately less time outdoors has likely contributed to opportunity structures that impede the development and sustaining of an active lifestyle. Part of the problem has been the construction and organization of environments, or the lack thereof, such as roadways, bikeways, green space, and community developments that deter people from playing, walking, or riding their bicycles, or at minimum do not facilitate such behaviour. An underlying issue is certainly the lack of a commitment by governments, as well as other organizations, to make an active society a priority in Canada.

BMI, Obesity, and Health

The relationship between body weight and health is also well established in the literature. A common measure used in the calculation of excess weight is body mass index (BMI), which is calculated as weight divided by height squared (BMI=kg/m2). There are various ranges of BMI considered to be healthy and unhealthy. These tend to be calculated for persons of a particular age and sex group. However, it should be noted that BMI calculations are not accurate for persons under age 20 and over age 64, and that pregnant women are omitted for obvious reasons. There is also some degree of controversy surrounding its validity and reliability as a measure of obesity, and, in turn, its causal link to diabetes, cardiovascular disease, and other chronic illnesses. One issue is the degree to which BMI correlates with accumulation of body fat in the midriff, which is a stronger correlate of cardiovascular disease. In addition, certain ethnic and racial groups may have different thresholds of risk associated with BMI than for the general population. However, BMI remains a standard and easily obtained indicator in the research literature on this topic. Additionally, although obesity is not a lifestyle per se, we consider it to be in large part an indicator of unhealthy eating habits and/or exercise levels.

According to the National Population Health Surveys (NPHS), a person with a BMI of 25 to 27 has some excess weight; a person with a BMI of 28 or above is considered overweight; and a person with a BMI of 30 or more is considered to be obese. This is consistent with most international research, although some researchers use a BMI of 27 and over as a definition of obesity. The choice of 30+ BMI as a cut-off for determining obesity in the present research is justified because it is obviously a stronger risk factor for chronic illness than using lower thresholds, the latter of which may include persons with borderline levels of fat. Based on 1998/99 NPHS data, 43% of Canadian women and 64% of men aged 20 to 64 had at least some excess weight; and 29% of women and 39% of men of that age group were overweight. Moreover, the obesity rate (persons with BMI levels of 30 or more) was found to be 14.8% for women and 15.5% for men aged 20 to 64 in 1998/99. In comparison, recent obesity rates in the U.S. are approximately 20%. Data from the Risk Factor Surveillance System in the U.S. show that over a 10-year period between 1985 and 1995, the rate of obesity (using the 30+ BMI definition) rose from 8.6% to 15.2% (CDC, 1996). Not only has the prevalence of obesity rates been on an incline since the early 1980s, but research indicates that telephone surveys may underestimate the actual rates by as much as 10% because they are based on self-reports (Cairney and Wade, 1997).

Obviously, obesity is related to eating patterns. Consuming larger portions of food and those containing higher amounts of saturated fats (low-density lipids) often found in fast foods (as compared to fruits, vegetables, and grains) result in weight excess (Binkley, Eales, and Jekanowski, 2000; Jeffery and French, 1998). Eating more fat than what our body requires, given our level of energy consumption, results in the storing of fat cells. It is recognized, however, that obesity may be the result of a genetic predisposition rather than lifestyle behaviour, but only in rare cases. In addition, diets associated with gaining weight may also lead to other deleterious effects on our health status. For instance, the consumption of food high in saturated fat (low density lipids) and trans fatty acids, such as deep-fried foods, leads to plaques and blockages in our cardiovascular system. Conversely, consuming more vegetables, fruits, and nuts can not only reduce weight but can also reduce serum lipids, which contribute to what is known as high cholesterol (Jenkins, Popovich, Kendall, Vidgen, Tariq, et al., 1997). Also, fats with high-density lipids, such as those in a Mediterranean diet using olive oil, and in fish (containing omega-3 fatty acids) have beneficial effects on our cardiovascular system.

In a large prospective U.S. study that followed 44,875 men aged 40 to 75 in 1985 for eight years, it was found that there were two main eating patterns associated with nonfatal myocardial infarction and fatal coronary heart disease, termed *hard CHD outcomes* (Hu, Rimm, Ascherio, Spiegelmann, and Willet, 2000). One is termed the *prudent pattern*, which is characterized by higher intake of vegetables, fruit, legumes, whole grains, fish, and poultry, whereas the other is called the *Western pattern*, which includes eating greater amounts of red meat, processed meat, refined grains, sweets and desserts, French fries, and high-fat dairy products. After adjusting for other risk factors of CHD, persons following the prudent diet exhibited a lower relative risk of hard CHD outcomes, and those who had a Western diet had higher relative risks. Another significant prospective study followed 22,043 Greek subjects aged 20 to 86 for a median of four years and compared persons who followed a Mediterranean diet versus a Western one (Hu, 2003). The researchers discovered that those following a traditional Greek diet extended their longevity by 25%. The Mediterranean diet consists of large amounts of vegetables, fruits, olives and olive oil, nuts, whole grains, moderate fish and dairy products, moderate amounts of red wine with most meals, and only small amounts of red meats. Following a Mediterranean-style diet has also been shown to improve symptoms associated with rheumatoid arthritis, including reduced inflammation, less pain, as well as increasing functional performance (Skokdstam, Hagfors, and Johansson, 2003). Thus, eating and nutrition patterns are multifaceted; moreover, there is ample evidence that they strongly influence our weight and our cardiovascular health, as well as a variety of additional health conditions.

Not surprisingly, there is also an inverse association between activity level and obesity level, but this association is not as strong as one might think and is overshadowed as a predictor by other lifestyle factors, in particular eating habits (Binkley et al., 2000). Furthermore, the major demographic and socioeconomic correlates of obesity in the literature include age, gender, socioeconomic status, and region. Unhealthy weight tends to peek in the early 50s and decrease as persons move into their elder years. In addition, higher obesity prevalence can be observed for men and lower SES (education, income, and occupation) persons, whereas lower rates occur among persons living in British Columbia and Quebec compared to the other provinces (Gilmore, 1999; Rabkin and Chen, 1997).

The growing prevalence of obesity has many serious consequences for the population health of Canadians. The cost of obesity in terms of health as well as productivity is enormous. For example, it has been estimated that the 1990 direct and indirect costs of excess weight in the U.S. were $46 billion and $23 billion, respectively (Wolf and Coldita, 1994). Persons who have excess weight are more likely to experience hypertension, heart disease, stroke, diabetes, breast cancer, and other chronic conditions (Cairney and Wade,

1998; Gilmore, 1999; Millar and Stephens, 1987; Rabkin and Chen, 1997; WHO, 1997). For example, in a secondary analysis of the 1994/95 National Population Health Survey, Cairney and Wade (1998) find that obese persons (compared to those of acceptable weight) are more than twice as likely to have diabetes and hypertension, and are significantly more likely to have arthritis, heart disease, and respiratory and stomach problems, and are more likely to report lower self-rated health. James, Young, Mustard, and Blanchard (1997) similarly analyse the 1994/95 NPHS finding that, among persons aged 45 to 64, 61% of those with diabetes were overweight (BMI = 28+) compared to only 38% of those without diabetes. Recent analysis of the subsequent 1996/97 NPHS by Gilmore (1999) has substantiated that obesity is associated with the above illnesses, as well as with asthma and back problems.

Thus, it can be observed that we are facing an obesity problem in North America, one that threatens to become worse, given current lifestyle patterns. Although the words 'crisis' and 'epidemic' have been used in the popular and academic literature to describe the recent trends in obesity, more research is needed to examine whether, and the degree to which, these lifestyle patterns indeed comprise a crisis or an epidemic. Moreover, whether the baby boom cohorts are contributing to this trend is as yet an unanswered question, and one that will receive considerable attention in this book.

Alcohol Consumption and Health

Drinking is part of most people's social life. About 77% of Canadians over the age of 15 consume alcoholic beverages (Single, Gliksman, and LeCavalier, 2000). In 1994, over half (58%) of adult Canadians reported that they were current drinkers (Statistics Canada, 1995b). Rates of heavy drinking are considerably lower, but depend on the definition used. The one used in the analyses in this book to represent heavy drinking is 14 or more alcoholic drinks per week for men and 12 or more for women. According to this definition, approximately 10% of Canadian adult men and 3% of adult women are heavy drinkers. Using a slightly different definition – 14 or more drinks per week for men, 9 or more drinks for women, with no more than 2 drinks on a given day – results in approximately 18% of the Canadian population exceeding this guideline. And these prevalence rates are based on self-reports, which tend to underestimate levels of alcohol consumption. There is also a link between drinking and smoking. The National Population Health Survey data indicate that about 25% of men and 16% of women are both smokers and current drinkers (Statistics Canada, 1995b).

Although most Canadians are moderate drinkers, a significant proportion of

Canadians are deemed to consume alcohol at levels that place them at risk for various health problems. Research pertaining to alcohol abuse demonstrates a number of deleterious effects on health (Andrews, 1988; Eckardt, Harford, Koelber, Parker, Rosenthal et al., 1981; Lamarche and Rootman, 1988; Statistics Canada, 1995a). These include motor vehicle accidents, cirrhosis of the liver, suicide, falls and other accidents, and breast cancer.

Single, Robson, Rehm, and Xie (1999) estimate that alcohol-attributed morbidity and mortality accounted for 3% of all deaths, 6% of the total years of potential life lost, 2% of hospitalizations, and 3% of total hospital days in Canada in 1992. However, the authors note that alcohol consumed in low or moderate amounts prevented at least as many deaths due to heart disease and stroke. Therefore, if health promotion programs reduce heavy drinking, and simultaneously encourage moderate drinking, the potential benefits to society could be enormous.

As with the previous lifestyle behaviours, there are many correlates of heavy drinking. One of the strongest of these is gender. Depending on the measures of heavy drinking or binge drinking used, men are between two and three times more likely to be in the high-risk group. Similar patterns are observed in the U.S. In addition, elevated rates of drinking and heavy drinking occur among young adults in their 20s; unemployed persons; high- and low-income persons; and persons of vulnerable populations, such as Aboriginals (Single et al., 1998). There is some truth to the stereotype of the drinker as a young single male. There is also extensive literature that establishes the strength of peer influence, health attitudes, and health beliefs pertaining to drinking on patterns of alcohol consumption. For example, believing in the relationship between drinking and cirrhosis proved to have a protective effect for heavy drinking among older persons (Ruchlin, 1997). Finally, there have been arguments put forth that the assiduous levels of stress in society have been pushing rates of drinking higher.

Clearly, alcohol consumption is part of our lifestyle as Canadians. Drinking can have both beneficial and harmful effects on our health and illness, depending on the amounts, types, and patterns of use. Like many of the other lifestyle behaviours, drinking is complex and associated with a large number of variables. But is heavy drinking becoming more prevalent over time, and is the baby boom generation contributing to these trends?

Multiplicity of Healthy Lifestyles

It is well established that people's healthy lifestyles shape their health trajectories. Although many health outcomes can be understood as a combination of a constellation of behaviours indicative of a healthy lifestyle, most research has focused on a singular factor. It is therefore advantageous to examine multiple health behaviours both from an individual and population health perspective, given that certain of these are correlated, whereas others are not. Indeed, some health behaviours appear to cluster together, whereas in other instances they may actually constrain one another. To make matters even more complicated, research suggests that improvement in one particular health behaviour does not necessarily mean improvement in others (Sobal, Revicki, and DeForge, 1992). It is instructive to examine some of the research that criss-crosses these issues.

There are definite associations among smoking, exercise, obesity, and heavy drinking – the major lifestyle behaviours investigated in this research. For example, persons who are overweight, drink heavily, or who smoke find it less easy to exercise and face a culmination of physical and psychological barriers that ultimately inhibit an active lifestyle. It is interesting, however, that obesity is most prevalent among former drinkers and former smokers, suggesting that eating may substitute for addictive behaviours and may itself comprise a type of addiction for certain individuals (Cairney and Wade, 1998; Gilmore, 1999). On the other hand, there are examples of correlations among various lifestyle behaviours.

For instance, eating patterns, and their result on body weight and body habatus, are also associated with a broader set of lifestyle behaviours, which likely coalesce. Research by Gillman et al. (2001) indicates that more sedentary individuals consume smaller amounts of foods and nutrients considered to be healthy, such as fruits and vegetables, fiber, calcium, folate, and vitamins A, C, and E, than do active individuals. They also establish that persons who are sedentary and consume a poor diet tend to congregate in groups with particular characteristics, such as low education, being unmarried, and being non-white. Perez (2002) adds to this literature by showing that, even accounting for the effects of health status and socio-demographic variables, smoking, physical activity, and BMI are independently associated with eating vegetables and fruits. Further, in the Seven Countries Study funded by the WHO, a combination of physical activity and diet-related variables accounted for 90% of the variance in body fat levels across seven different countries (Kromhout, Bloemberg, Seidell, Nissinen, and Menotti, 2001).

There also may be additive and interactive effects among lifestyle factors. It has been demonstrated that being overweight and inactive pose cumulative risks for diabetes among Canadians aged 45 to 64 (James et al., 1997). Additionally, the risk of cardiovascular disease increases exponentially with the constellation of risk factors present, including smoking, inactivity, obesity, heavy drinking, and diabetes (Grundy, 1999; Johansen, Nargundkar, Nair, Taylor, and ElSaadany, 1998; Neaton and Wentworth, 1992). It is therefore imperative that we not only recognize the interconnectedness of lifestyle behaviours, but that we also consider several key ones in any assessment of the health of Canadians. Given the research questions guiding this book, the focus will be on examining patterns of change in the rate of each of the four selected health behaviours, rather than analyses of particular combinations, such as persons who are sedentary and obese. However, efforts will be made to compare and contrast the patterns across lifestyles in an effort to synthesize the results.

Taken together, the substantial body of literature on lifestyle behaviours provides compelling evidence for the preventive and rehabilitative influence of several notable health behaviours. On the other side of the coin, there are patterns in lifestyles that are unhealthy among certain groups. In particular, males, persons with lower education and income, and those living in particular regions tend to engage in more unhealthy lifestyles. Availability of a set of lifestyle measures for multiple, cross-sectional, national Canadian data sets allows for examination of several major ones: smoking, physical activity/ exercise, body weight (body mass index), and alcohol consumption. These will be investigated along with other key variables such as gender, education, and income, and subsequently compared against trends in health status and health utilization for specific age groups in order to address questions pertaining to comparative health patterns of baby boomers and previous generations.

5

Data Sources and Data Analyses

The Selection of Health Surveys

The type of age-period-cohort analysis employed in this book is based on sequential cross-sectional surveys (Wolinsky, 1993). Standard measures across multiple survey dates are required, typically a minimum of three (Glenn, 1977). Extending research conducted by Kendall, Lipskie, and MacEachern (1997), a total of 27 national Canadian surveys that incorporated questions on health and related variables of interest were identified for possible inclusion in this research. Each survey was evaluated in terms of availability of data covering the four key domains for this research: lifestyle health behaviours, chronic conditions, health utilization, and socio-economic variables. The potential for standard measure construction and the potential for disaggregation into age-sex cohorts was considered for each data set. Based on this analysis, a set of standardized measures were found for six national health surveys covering an average of 22 years – between 1978/79 and 2000/01. These include the 1978/79 Canada Health Survey, 1985 and 1990 Health Promotion Surveys, 1994/95 and 1998/99 National Population Health Surveys, and the 2000/01 Canadian Community Health Survey. It will be observed that each of these surveys reflects a particular conceptual framing of health and illness that was popular during the survey period.

All six of the surveys included in this book are large national surveys of the non-institutional Canadian population, excluding residents of the territories, Native reserves, and remote areas. Although both weighted and unweighted data are analysed, only the weighted data will be presented. Weighted data converts age-sex sub-sample groups to their respective population sizes, given the complex stratification and clustering designs used to sample.

The 1978/79 Canada Health Survey

The Canadian Health Survey (CHS) is one of the earliest national surveys that provides comprehensive data on health status and health behaviours. The survey was conducted by Statistics Canada and Health and Welfare Canada and was collected between May 1978 and March 1979. The CHS has a sample size of 12,218 households (Chen and Millar, 2000). There were several components to the survey. The Interviewer Administered Questionnaire (IAQ) involved the collection of self-reported chronic conditions and activity restriction for all members of the household from a target household member. The Lifestyle and Health Questionnaire (LHQ) was administered to household members aged 15 and over. Members of a subset of households in the interview component were also asked to participate in obtaining information for the Physical Measures Questionnaire (PMQ), which entailed obtaining measurements of blood pressure, cardio-respiratory fitness, height, weight, and skin fold of household members aged 2 and over, as well as blood samples from a smaller subset of persons aged 3 and over. The response rates were 86% for the IAQ (10,571 households), 89% for the LHQ (23,791 respondents), and 72% for the PMQ (6,131 respondents).

The 1978/79 Canada Health Survey data are shown in Table 5.1 by five-year age group and sex. Each sample has been weighted to the total Canadian population, and the actual numbers and percentages are shown separately for males and females, as well as for the total population. The 70 and over ages were collapsed into one group because of the unavailability of further disaggregation in the Public Use Data Files, due to the fact that certain data are protected for privacy issues in instances in which sub-sample numbers become small. It is recognized that under the recent data liberation exercise of Statistics Canada that the Master Files are available through the Research Data Centres. However, further age breakdowns above 70 are not conducted in this analysis because it would cause a significant decrease in sub-sample sizes by sex and other variables, and therefore would result in large sub-sample variability and sampling error. The percentages for males and females are row percentages, which give the proportion of the total that males and females contribute for each five-year cohort, and the total weighted population. For example, Table 5.1 shows that males made up 49.1% and females comprised 50.9% of the total population in 1978/79. The column total percentages give the proportion that each five-year age group contributes to the total population. At the youngest ages, for example, the 15- to 19-year cohort made up 13.3% of the total 15 and over, non-institutional, non-reserve population. At the oldest, the 70 and over group comprised 7.2%.

Table 5.1
1978/79 Canada Health Survey

Age Group	Males N	%	Females N	%	Total N	%
15–19	1,187,236	50.9	1,145,667	49.1	2,332,903	13.3
20–24	1,106,355	50.0	1,108,335	50.0	2,214,690	12.7
25–29	990,479	49.6	1,005,547	50.4	1,996,026	11.4
30–34	904,116	50.0	905,727	50.0	1,809,843	10.3
35–39	716,673	50.1	714,482	49.9	1,431,155	8.2
40–44	618,645	50.1	616,482	49.9	1,235,127	7.1
45–49	623,829	50.3	616,815	49.7	1,240,644	7.1
50–54	590,009	49.1	611,132	50.9	1,201,141	6.9
55–59	532,150	48.0	577,535	52.0	1,109,685	6.3
60–64	427,930	47.5	473,395	52.5	901,325	5.2
65–69	356,939	46.8	406,250	53.2	763,189	4.4
70+	529,708	42.2	726,111	57.8	1,255,819	7.2
Total	8,584,069	49.1	8,907,478	50.9	17,491,547	100.0

Note: Numbers are weighted to the population.

The 1985 and 1990 Health Promotion Surveys

The 1985 and 1990 Health Promotion Surveys (HPS) provide extensive information on the health promotion activities of Canadians. The development of the Health Promotion Directorate in 1982, with a new mandate to foster a national health promotion program, led to the planning and implementation of these surveys. Thus, the 1985 and 1990 HPSs were designed to provide important information on the health promotion behaviours of Canadians for the purpose of supporting this national programmatic effort. Several substantive areas are covered in these surveys, including exercise, nutrition, smoking, alcohol use, drug use, safety, mental health, and sexual behaviour. The major conceptual frameworks upon which the HPSs were constructed include the Precede Model (Green, 1980), the Health Belief Model (Rosenstock, 1974), and the models underlying the Canadian Health Survey and the Canadian Fitness Survey. These emphasize both the health behaviours and the intentions, attitudes, and beliefs underlying health behaviour.

The 1985 and 1990 HPSs relied on telephone interviewing techniques as part of the new generation of survey interviewing. The target population for both the 1985 and 1990 HPSs was persons aged 15 and over. The samples were

Table 5.2 1985
Health Promotion Survey

Age Group	Males N	%	Females N	%	Total N	%
15–19	1,000,748	51.1	956,048	48.9	1,956,796	10.0
20–24	1,202,223	50.6	1,174,152	49.4	2,376,375	12.1
25–29	1,090,439	49.2	1,125,990	50.8	2,216,429	11.3
30–34	1,134,909	50.2	1,124,360	49.8	2,259,269	11.5
35–39	1,015,850	52.8	909,478	47.2	1,925,328	9.8
40–44	753,161	47.0	850,840	53.0	1,604,001	8.2
45–49	601,086	51.1	575,282	48.9	1,176,368	6.0
50–54	662,171	49.3	681,887	50.7	1,344,058	6.9
55–59	617,691	52.3	563,713	47.7	1,181,404	6.0
60–64	489,888	43.5	635,042	56.5	1,124,930	5.7
65–69	457,414	46.0	536,918	54.0	994,332	5.1
70+	596,989	41.1	854,811	58.9	1,451,800	7.4
Total	9,622,569	49.1	9,988,521	50.9	19,611,090	100.0

Note: Numbers are weighted to the population.

drawn from the Canadian Labour Force Surveys, and resulted in 11,181 completed interviews for the 1985 HPS and 13,793 for the 1990 HPS. Response rates were slightly over 80% in both surveys.

Table 5.2 shows the 1985 HPS by five-year age group and sex in the same manner as above. It can be seen that in 1985, 15- to 19-year-olds only comprised 10% of the total population in that year, a drop of 3.3% from 1978/ 79, whereas the 70 and over age group increased slightly to 7.4% (from 7.2%), revealing the beginning signs of population aging in Canada. Table 5.3 shows identical data for the 1990 HPS. A further drop is observed for persons aged 15 to 19, where it is noted that they made up only 8.9% of the total population, reflecting continued drops in fertility in the 1970s. The 70 and over age group rose more rapidly due to population aging, from 7.4% in 1985 to 8.7% in 1990.

The National Population Health Surveys

The National Population Health Surveys (NPHS) began in 1994/95 and have been repeated in 1996/97 and 1998/99. This study only uses the 1994/95 and 1998/99 surveys. The NPHS collects information on a variety of health components much like the earlier surveys. However, the NPHS adds another

Table 5.3
1990 Health Promotion Survey

Age Group	Males N	%	Females N	%	Total N	%
15–19	943,540	51.2	898,713	48.8	1,842,253	8.9
20–24	1,002,404	50.7	973,126	49.3	1,975,530	9.6
25–29	1,174,924	49.8	1,182,014	50.2	2,356,938	11.4
30–34	1,170,458	49.6	1,190,891	50.4	2,361,349	11.4
35–39	1,073,253	49.5	1,096,346	50.5	2,169,599	10.5
40–44	981,909	49.8	990,168	50.2	1,972,077	9.6
45–49	775,722	50.2	769,848	49.8	1,545,570	7.5
50–54	627,313	49.7	635,459	50.3	1,262,772	6.1
55–59	592,371	49.5	605,545	50.5	1,197,916	5.8
60–64	550,190	48.2	591,072	51.8	1,141,262	5.5
65–69	467,350	45.5	559,021	54.5	1,026,371	5.0
70+	737,775	41.2	1,053,967	58.8	1,791,742	8.7
Total	10,097,209	48.9	10,546,170	51.1	20,643,379	100.0

Note: Numbers are weighted to the population.

conceptual model – the Population Health Framework – which, as discussed earlier, emphasizes determinants of health that cover a broad spectrum of variables.

A special component of the NPHS sampled individuals living in institutions; however, these persons will be omitted from the analyses. In addition, a battery of supplemental questions were asked of the core sample of longitudinal respondents (about 15,000 individuals who were identified for re-interview). The supplement includes questions on several topics: individual diets and eating habits, breast feeding, attitudes of mothers about alcohol consumption during pregnancy, knowledge and attitudes about preventive sexual health, and opinions about the quality of health care services.

The 1994/95 NPHS

The 1994/95 NPHS is composed of 19,600 households drawn randomly from the Labour Force Survey sampling frame and has a response rate of 88 (Statistics Canada, 1995b). One individual from each household was randomly selected for an in-depth interview and a subset of information was collected on each household. The survey includes questions related to the following key

Table 5.4
1994/95 National Population Health Survey

Age Group	Males		Females		Total	
	N	%	N	%	N	%
15–19	1,057,275	51.7	989,001	48.3	2,046,276	9.0
20–24	837,416	48.1	902,131	51.9	1,739,547	7.7
25–29	1,081,492	50.5	1,058,399	49.5	2,139,891	9.5
30–34	1,256,270	48.0	1,359,332	52.0	2,615,602	11.6
35–39	1,321,761	50.9	1,272,499	49.1	2,594,260	11.5
40–44	1,152,329	50.8	1,117,744	49.2	2,270,073	10.0
45–49	1,020,450	51.9	944,966	48.1	1,965,416	8.7
50–54	796,597	51.8	742,047	48.2	1,538,644	6.8
55–59	601,308	46.8	684,576	53.2	1,285,884	5.7
60–64	551,075	46.9	624,841	53.1	1,175,916	5.2
65–69	523,806	47.4	581,993	52.6	1,105,799	4.9
70+	874,814	40.8	1,270,354	59.2	2,145,168	9.5
Total	11,074,593	49.0	11,547,883	51.0	22,622,476	100.0

Note: Numbers are weighted to the population.

areas: health determinants (including socio-economic status, smoking, alcohol use, physical activities, disabilities, self-esteem, mastery, social support, etc.); health status (including perceived health, mental health, chronic conditions, the general health status index, and activity restriction); and use of health services (visits to traditional and non-traditional health care providers, and drug and medication use).

Table 5.4 presents the weighted five-year age and sex breakdown of the Canadian population. Little change is seen in the proportion (9%) of the population that the 15- to 19-year-olds comprise. However, the proportion contributed by the 70 and over group increased to 9.5% as population aging continued to rise steadily.

The 1998/99 NPHS

The 1998/99 NPHS is similar to the 1994/95 version except that it contains a panel component for a sub-sample. Since we are interested in health trends across several cross-sectional surveys, we employ the cross-sectional component of the 1998/99 NPHS – a sample of 14,682. Table 5.5 shows the weighted five-year age and sex breakdown of the Canadian population. And again, the

Table 5.5
1998/99 National Population Health Survey

Age Group	Males		Females		Total	
	N	%	N	%	N	%
15–19	1,092,483	51.0	1,047,889	49.0	2,140,372	9.0
20–24	970,659	50.3	959,127	49.7	1,929,786	8.1
25–29	933,519	51.5	879,364	48.5	1,812,883	7.6
30–34	1,101,079	47.6	1,210,877	52.4	2,311,956	9.7
35–39	1,363,175	49.3	1,400,301	50.7	2,763,476	11.6
40–44	1,377,633	51.8	1,282,302	48.2	2,659,935	11.2
45–49	1,006,933	47.6	1,109,710	52.4	2,116,643	8.9
50–54	946,619	50.6	922,602	49.4	1,869,221	7.9
55–59	723,445	52.8	647,266	47.2	1,370,711	5.8
60–64	629,603	47.7	691,011	52.3	1,320,614	5.6
65–69	494,798	45.0	605,355	55.0	1,100,153	4.6
70+	1,022,841	42.8	1,364,619	57.2	2,387,460	10.0
Total	11,662,787	49.0	12,120,423	51.0	23,783,210	100.0

Note: Numbers are weighted to the population.

15- to 19-year-olds make up 9% of the total target population, but the 70 and over age group reaches 10%. Adding this percentage to the 4.6% of the total population comprising persons aged 65 to 69, we observe an elderly population of 14.6% of the total population of Canada in 1998/99.

The 2000/01 Community Health Survey

In 2000/01 the NPHS was changed to the Canadian Community Health Survey (CCHS). This survey was also developed to provide data pertaining to health determinants, health status, and health system utilization at the sub-provincial, provincial, and national levels (Béland, 2002). The CCHS has a total sample of 130,000, which provides opportunities for analyses of health data at a number of levels. The health topics covered in this survey are the same as those in the NPHS, but also include more detailed variables than what have been used previously. Overall, the CCHS provides excellent data for this type of analysis and is the most comprehensive and representative health survey of the general population in Canadian history. Table 5.6 presents the five-year age data showing slight increases among persons aged 65 to 69 and 70 and over compared to the 1998/99 NPHS.

Table 5.6
2000/01 Canadian Community Health Survey

	Males		Females		Total	
Age Group	N	%	N	%	N	%
15–19	1,091,375	51.2	1,040,623	48.8	2,131,998	8.7
20–24	1,073,330	50.8	1,039,238	49.2	2,112,568	8.6
25–29	1,013,359	50.5	992,661	49.5	2,006,020	8.2
30–34	1,093,262	50.6	1,065,727	49.4	2,158,989	8.8
35–39	1,276,546	49.3	1,311,096	50.7	2,587,642	10.5
40–44	1,358,016	50.1	1,349,953	49.9	2,707,969	11.0
45–49	1,166,274	49.2	1,203,159	50.8	2,369,433	9.6
50–54	1,020,289	49.7	1,031,657	50.3	2,051,946	8.3
55–59	800,472	50.5	784,753	49.5	1,585,225	6.4
60–64	604,019	48.5	640,592	51.5	1,244,611	5.1
65–69	549,536	47.7	602,020	52.3	1,151,556	4.7
70+	1,044,482	41.9	1,448,774	58.1	2,493,256	10.1
Total	12,090,960	49.1	12,510,253	50.9	24,601,213	100.0

Note: Numbers are weighted to the population.

Selection of Health and Social Variables

The health and social data selected for examination across the seven national health surveys between 1978/79 and 2000/01 coincide with the four primary domains, and include (1) lifestyle health behaviours – smoking, exercise, BMI, and alcohol consumption; (2) chronic health conditions – number of chronic conditions, rates for hypertension, diabetes, and arthritis; (3) health utilization – doctor visits; and (4) SES measures – education and income, region, and foreign-born status. The precise measurement of each of these variables is discussed in conjunction with the results.

Age of Baby Boomers at Each Survey Date

As can be seen in Table 5.7, the birth cohorts of the baby boom generation range from 1946 to 1965. The survey dates include 1978/79, 1985, 1990, 1994/95, 1998/99, and 2000/01. The 1998/99 survey data are used only in selected analyses because they were collected only two years apart from the other two adjacent surveys and therefore are not useful for the five-year age-period-cohort analyses. Persons at the front end of the baby boom generation

Table 5.7
Age of Baby Boomers at Each Survey Date

Year Born	Survey Year					
	1978	1985	1990	1994	1998	2000
1946	32	39	44	48	52	54
1947	31	38	43	47	51	53
1948	30	37	42	46	50	52
1949	29	36	41	45	49	51
1950	28	35	40	44	48	50
1951	27	34	39	43	47	49
1952	26	33	38	42	46	48
1953	25	32	37	41	45	47
1954	24	31	36	40	44	46
1955	23	30	35	39	43	45
1956	22	29	34	38	42	44
1957	21	28	33	37	41	43
1958	20	27	32	36	40	42
1959	19	26	31	35	39	41
1960	18	25	30	34	38	40
1961	17	24	29	33	37	39
1962	16	23	28	32	36	38
1963	15	22	27	31	35	37
1964	14	21	26	30	34	36
1965	13	20	25	29	33	35

were born in 1946 and were aged 32 in 1978 and 54 in 2000 (see Table 5.7). Someone born in the middle of the baby boom generation would be born in about 1955, and would be aged 23 in 1978 and 45 in 2000. A person at the tail end of the baby boom generation would be born in 1965, and thus only 13 years of age in 1978 and 35 years of age in 2000. Since the 1978/79 Canada Health Survey collected information on individuals aged 15 and over, the 1964 and 1965 birth cohorts (aged 13 and 14, respectively, in 1978) cannot be included in our tables and figures until the second survey date, in 1985.

Table 5.8 presents the approximate age range of the four, five-year birth cohorts comprising the 20-year baby boom generation. Those born between 1946 and 1950 were aged 28 to 32 in 1978, and were aged 50 to 54 in 2000. Those at the other extreme, born between 1961 and 1965 were aged 13 to 17 in 1978 and 35 to 39 in 2000. These align nicely with the typical five-year age groupings used in demographic analyses; for example, 15 to 19, 20 to 24, 25 to 29, and so on.

Table 5.8
Age Range of Baby Boomers at Each Survey Date

	Survey Year					
Year Born	1978	1985	1990	1994	1998	2000
1950–1946	28–32	35–39	40–44	44–48	48–52	50–54
1955–1951	23–28	30–34	35–39	39–43	43–47	45–49
1960–1956	18–22	25–29	30–34	34–38	38–42	40–44
1965–1961	13–17	20–24	25–29	29–33	33–37	35–39

Age-Period-Cohort Analyses

The proposed research will use sequential cross-sectional analyses of standard cohort tables (also known as synthetic cohorts). This type of research is typically called cohort analyses, or age-period-cohort analyses. This analytic technique is well suited to explore the health dynamics of the baby boom generation using the survey data available for this research, the cohorts comprising it, and for comparisons with other birth cohorts and generations (Glenn, 1977). Our use of sequential cross-sectional surveys will be restricted to assessments of aggregate-level change rather than intra-individual change, the latter of which requires panel data; that is, information on the same individuals at different survey points. In order to conduct this type of analysis, intervals between ages and survey points must be regularized – approximately equal (Wolinsky, 1993).

The initial step in conducting age-period-cohort analyses of sequential cross-sectional data is the construction of age-sex-specific cohort tables. The percentage of persons reporting a specified level or category of a health variable (e.g., smoking, obesity, diabetes, doctor visits, etc.) is calculated for each age group and by sex for all survey periods. The age groups (e.g., 5-year age groups) need to correspond as closely as possible to the separation of survey dates (e.g., 5 years apart), so that one can compare time trends for a particular age group that correspond to the length between the surveys. In the present research, five-year age groups are used. Due to the possibility of different sampling errors across age, sex, and survey, standard 95% confidence intervals are calculated for all of the population estimates, and these are used to make decisions about restricting the analyses for those variables/age-groups deemed to be susceptible to this problem (Wolinsky, 1993). Sub-samples in which there is high sampling error also have high sampling variability and therefore large confidence intervals, indicating that the population estimate can be variable across other sub-samples of this size. However, the magnitude of the surveys used in these analyses tend to be large, which shrinks the confidence intervals significantly, and therefore makes the estimates more robust and minimizes this error (Wolinsky, 1993). The majority of the analyses are based on large subgroups that tend to be accurate population estimates within a range of a percentage point or two. Analyses in which data are restricted because of high sampling variability are noted.

Let us turn to a description of age-period-cohort analyses and how they can be estimated in sequential cross-sectional survey tables. We use the term *estimation*, because analyses of age and time trends in cross-sectional, or even panel data, entail complex combinations of age, period, and cohort (age by period interaction) effects that are not easily separated (Palmore, 1978; Selvin, 1996), especially when interactions among them exist. For this reason, our purpose for using these methods is to identify prominent and substantively important patterns pertaining to lifestyle behaviours and the health of Canadians, rather than attempt to separate each effect in a concise manner. This will allow us to determine whether and to what degree recent changes in the health dynamics of baby boomers are better or worse than what we would have anticipated if they aged much like prior cohorts of individuals. Furthermore, in a prospective sense, we will also be able to ascertain whether the progression of health outcomes for baby boomers will pose a greater or lesser problem for population health, and, ultimately, for our health care system. And, finally, this analysis will allow for identification of trends specific to other key age and sex groups.

We illustrate the age-period-cohort analytic strategy in Table 5.9. Historical, or *period*, influences can be estimated by comparing health characteristics of the same age group across survey time periods. In other words, we can compare across the rows for a particular age group, as shown by the shaded area designated as A in Table 5.9. For example, comparisons of the percentage of persons who smoke could be made for persons of the same five-year age group (e.g., persons aged 15–19) at all relevant survey time intervals. This is repeated for all other age groups under examination by also reading across the rows in the table. These comparisons control for chronological aging and afford an opportunity for identification of any significant increases or decreases in prevalence rates for a specific age group at different periods anchored to the survey dates.

However, seldom are these period trends 'pure' effects. Indeed, they may include interactions with cohort effects, since individuals may be differentially affected by historical events at different points in their lives (Selvin, 1996; Wolinsky, 1993). For instance, a larger decline in the smoking prevalence

Table 5.9
Illustration of Age, Period, Cohort Analytic Strategy
Male Smoking Prevalence (per cent)

| Age Group | Survey Year | | | | |
	1980	1985	1990	1995	2000
15–19	35	24	20	19	18
20–24	51	35	32	27	29
25–29	49	37	35	32	30
30–34	43	37	34	35	29
35–39	46	33	37	31	28
40–44	49	33	34	35	31
45–49	52	37	28	30	30
50–54	46	37	30	27	25
55–59	40	28	34	27	22
60–64	40	28	26	23	18
65–69	39	18	21	14	16
70+	28	18	15	14	9
Total	44	31	30	27	25

A. Period effects + interactions on smoking prevalence for males aged 15–19.
B. Cohort effects + interactions on smoking prevalence for the year 2000.
C. Age effects + interactions for males born between 1961 and 1965.

among younger persons over the last few years compared to other age groups could reflect the differential influence of recent anti-smoking campaigns on normative expectations surrounding smoking, a period-cohort interaction. In the hypothetical example in Table 5.9, it can be observed that the smoking rate for males 15 to19 dropped from 35% in 1980 to 24% in 1985, 20% in 1990, 19% in 1995, and 18% in 2000. Thus, in this example, teenage smoking rates for males dropped by almost half between 1980 and 2000, and the greatest drop in its prevalence occurred between 1980 and 1985. An analysis of period effects also identifies whether patterns observed for one age group is replicated for others. Patterns that are repeated for a number of age groups are indicative of substantively important period effects. In addition, it is informative to report period changes in prevalence rates for the total population. This is accomplished by examining rates across the bottom row of the table, designated *Total*. For example, the bottom row in Table 5.9 shows that the smoking rate for all Canadian males dropped from 44% in 1978.79 to 25% in 2000/01.

Cohort membership effects can be determined by observing the *inter*cohort changes that occur in a health variable for representative samples (or sub-samples) of persons aged 15 to 19, 20 to 24, and so on (Wolinsky, 1993). For example, smoking rates among age groups for a particular survey year can be investigated, as in our hypothetical example in Table 5.9, where the shaded area designated as B represents cohort effects in the year 2000. This allows for comparison of the smoking rates of persons of different birth cohorts in 2000. For example, the smoking rate was 18% for persons 15 to19 in 2000, but rises to about 30% for persons in their 20s and 30s, peaks at 35% for persons 45 to 49, and declines thereafter (see B, Table 5.9). Again, changes in rates that are repeated across different periods (surveys) may be indicative, for example, of the influence of a rise in education over time that may differentially influence expectations regarding smoking among successive cohorts. It should be noted that, intuitively, one might consider that smoking rates by a five-year age group for a specific year is indicative of smoking over the 'life cycle' – or a type of 'aging' effect. However, these rates are composed of representative samples of persons of different birth cohorts who are not necessarily going to follow the same 'aging' trajectory in a health variable. Furthermore, as in the above example, there may be interactions with period effects.

In this sense, period and cohort effects cannot fully explain different health behaviours and health statuses observed in a population, since there are also aging-related changes in individuals as they mature, termed *age* effects. Age effects can be estimated by examining *intra*cohort differences over time. For example, using five-year age-sex tables as shown in Table 5.9, we can compare percentages of persons who smoke regularly in a representative sample of persons aged 15 to19 in 1980 with persons aged 20 to 24 in 1985, 25 to 29 in 1990, 30 to 34 in 1995, and 35 to 39 in 2000. This is accomplished by reading diagonally down and to the right of each table, as shown in the shaded area designated as C in Table 5.9. Here, smoking rates among persons of the same birth cohort can be examined as they age, and therefore focus attention on aging effects of a specific birth cohort over the specified time period. These control for the effects of different birth cohorts by examining each one separately, but once again may also reflect interactions with period and cohort. As in the other examples, this process would be repeated for all remaining cohorts. Patterns that are replicated across different birth cohorts would be highlighted.

Although these descriptions appear straightforward, there are a number of limitations with this type of analysis. Only those that are not mitigated by the use of large survey data will be discussed. *Compositional change* is the problem that occurs due to attrition from the death of individuals that may create a bias, in the same manner that mortality influences internal validity of experimental designs (Wolinksy, 1993). For example, if the healthiest people survive, then the comparisons across time periods are not fair. This problem is more serious for elderly groups and is further reason why more detailed age breakdowns are not used beyond age 70.

A second and more serious obstacle to interpretation of age, period, and cohort effects is the problem of *identification*, which refers to the statistical confounding of age, period, and cohort due to interactions among them (Glenn, 1989). Simply put, identification of 'pure' age, period, or cohort effects are tenuous because in reality they are not independent of one another. For instance, making row comparisons to uncover age effects also invariably includes cohort and period effects because one is comparing different birth cohorts at different points in time. This underscores the complexity of this type of analysis, and the need to carefully interpret results against current knowledge of age, period, and cohort trends linked to a health variable (Palmore, 1978). Indeed, the more one knows about these effects beforehand, based on theoretical axioms and other research findings, the easier will be the interpretation.

For example, the introduction of the *ParticipAction* program in 1971, which grew in intensity and awareness throughout the 1980s and 1990s, probably affected younger persons at that time more than elderly ones, because the former would be in the more mutable stage of developing patterns of exercise behaviour. Also, economic indicators, such as fluctuations in the gross domestic product (GDP), can influence the health of age groups differently depending on their age when exposed to those swings. These are examples of period-cohort interactions. According to Wolinsky (1993), Palmore (1978), and Glenn (1977), the solutions to these complexities are (1) to make explicit theoretical expectations before the analyses; (2) to look for monotonic and repeated patterns in the data; and (3) to adopt high standards in accepting interactions among age, period, and cohort effects. While there have been statistical developments using multivariate techniques while making assumptions about either age, period, or cohort effects, the utility of these techniques have been seriously questioned (Selvin, 1996). Moreover, these methods are not appropriate for this type of analysis. We therefore rely on conventional age- period-cohort methods, and adopt the approaches described above using sequential cross-sectional tables and graphical representations of these tables.

In keeping with the recommendations above, it is hypothesized that period and cohort effects will be stronger than age effects in accounting for changes in health behaviours. This is because age effects, in general, tend to be slower to change than the other two. With respect to interactions among these components, it is also hypothesized that changes in economic conditions will have more adverse outcomes for the health of older baby boomers, born between

1946 and 1955, than among the younger boomers, born between 1956 and 1965, because the former would be in their career phase of employment. Furthermore, the identification of macro social change trends in GDP, income distribution, educational attainment, number of physicians per population, and major policies regarding the provision of health care services over the approximately 22- year period under study will be instrumental for the identification of hypotheses linked to interpretation of age, period, and cohort effects, and will help to deal with the complexities of this problem (Glenn, 1989).

The relationships discussed above are shown in both table and graphical form so that visual comparisons can be made among cohorts, different health domains, and social change indicators. The values for each period are plotted using different symbols so that trends can be observed. Also, the plots for the baby boom cohorts are set apart. Inspection of the plotted patterns will provide an opportunity to reflect upon the main research questions and to identify the most salient healthy lifestyle trajectories.

The five primary surveys used (1978/79; 1985; 1990; 1994/95; and 2000/01) are not equally spaced at five-year intervals; however, they have been selected because they are close as possible to five-year periods and contain the variables of interest with standard measurement. It will be necessary to make only minor adjustments to compare rates to make fair comparisons across the periods. It is useful to repeat that all data used for this research have been weighted, and individual age-sex-specific cohorts have been checked for adequate sampling variability associated with sub-sample sizes, including the calculation of confidence intervals around population parameters.

We begin with an age-period-cohort analysis of the four major lifestyle behaviours, or their outcomes in the case of obesity: smoking, unhealthy exercise levels, obesity, and heavy drinking. This is followed by a separate analysis of chronic illness and utilization data in a subsequent chapter. Additionally, the baby boomer cohorts are specifically focused upon in separate chapters, and include variations by SES, region, and foreign-born status.

6

Changes in Healthy Lifestyles for the Canadian Population

In this chapter, patterns of healthy lifestyles are analysed for the adult Canadian population in order to identify age, period, and cohort changes in these important dimensions of health behaviour. While the focus of this book is on the baby boom generation, it is first necessary to examine the total population in this type of analysis before turning specifically to the boomers in subsequent chapters. This is because identification of particular age-time patterns necessitates demonstration of repeated trends. Furthermore, analysis of the complete adult Canadian population affords opportunity to investigate various age-sex groups as they move along the age escalator, which will provide a backdrop upon which a focused study of the baby boom generation can be made.

As detailed in the previous chapter, we will undertake period analyses by comparing the prevalence rates for the lifestyle behaviours for the same five-year age- and sex-specific groups across the survey dates (period effects). These are combined with *inter*cohort changes (cohort effects) within surveys to identify whether there are replicated patterns in health dynamics for the various birth cohorts or whether some appear to be shifting more than others. *Intra*cohort analyses (aging effects) are conducted in a subsequent analysis by following specific age cohorts for each of the survey periods and comparing them. We supplement these investigations with identification of key historical events and make assumptions about their differential impact on age-time trends. Our cohort analysis will also entail comparing, contrasting, and integrating these patterns to pinpoint interactions among these effects (Giele and Elder, 1998). Finally, gender comparisons are presented separately, since age-time trends in these lifestyle behaviours vary by sex.

How Have Patterns of Smoking Changed?

Tables 6.1 and 6.2 show the percentage of the population who are regular smokers (by five-year age group) for each of the surveys with separate tables for males and females. It was necessary to group persons aged 70 and over because of sample restrictions and sub-sample size issues. Figures 6.1 and 6.2 display these tabular data in graphical form for visual inspection and presentation of the most significant trends. Each survey is presented with a distinct line pattern, and the baby boom generation cohorts are identified for preliminary exploration. We report point differences in rates (i.e., absolute percentage differences), as well as relative percentage changes in the rates (i.e., percentage changes between two time periods).

Improved Smoking Patterns for Men

A consistent decline has occurred in the prevalence rate of regular smoking over the time period studied. The bottom row in Table 6.1 indicates that the percentage of the total Canadian male population aged 15 and over who smoke regularly dropped from 43.9% in 1978/79 to 30.6% in 1985, 29.8% in 1990, 27.4% in 1994/95, and 24.6% in 2000/01. This amounts to a reduction in the rate of smoking by almost one-half over this 22-year span. As can be observed in Figure 6.1, the most rapid decreases occurred between 1978/79 and 1985. Since the intervals between surveys are not perfectly equal, especially the first and last surveys, which are separated by an average of 6.5 and 6 years, respectively, comparisons should be made with caution. However, even taking into account these period lengths between surveys through interpolation (linear adjustment to a standard five-year period), the decline in smoking is still most pronounced between the first two survey dates. These period patterns coincide with the initiation of anti-smoking campaigns in Canada and the United States in the late 1970s and early 1980s.

Examination of the individual five-year age groups over the survey dates reveals other noteworthy trends. First, there is an inverted U-shaped curve to smoking rates across the age groups for each time period, such that the middle-aged groups exhibit the highest rates (see Figure 6.1). Second, the shape of this pattern softens over time periods for particular age groups. For instance, the drop in smoking between 1978/79 and 2000/01 has been greater for males aged 45 to 49 than for those aged 30 to 34. This is indicative of some age-period and period-cohort interaction. Third, the smoking rates for the latest period (2000/01) are the lowest for all age groups other than teenagers. In

Table 6.1
Percentage of Canadian Population Regular Smokers* by 5-Year Age Groups, Males, 1978/79–2000/01

Age Group	Survey									
	1978/79 CHS		1985 HPS*		1990 HPS		1994/95 NPHS		2000/01 CCHS	
	N	%	N	%	N	%	N	%	N	%
15–19	383,378	34.7	237,663	23.9	187,173	20.0	196,437	18.6	190,979	17.7
20–24	540,656	50.7	417,232	34.7	323,253	32.2	222,628	26.6	311,130	29.1
25–29	466,422	48.9	385,394	37.3	407,380	34.7	350,244	32.4	304,146	30.1
30–34	370,837	43.2	443,691	37.3	403,194	34.4	442,941	35.2	321,407	29.5
35–39	317,195	45.9	355,019	33.3	394,914	36.9	410,893	31.1	358,628	28.2
40–44	286,153	49.0	237,576	33.3	334,404	34.0	399,645	34.7	413,265	30.6
45–49	302,128	52.0	284,076	37.0	216,549	27.9	309,300	30.4	344,948	29.7
50–54	256,447	46.2	176,360	37.0	185,670	29.6	217,483	27.3	251,657	24.7
55–59	202,740	40.4	185,499	28.2	197,076	33.6	160,958	26.7	174,897	21.9
60–64	162,012	40.2	129,394	28.2	144,528	26.5	126,857	23.0	109,951	18.3
65–69	130,532	39.7	102,959	18.4	97,004	20.8	74,807	14.3	87,874	16.0
70+	132,531	28.4	85,476	18.4	113,902	15.4	125,875	14.4	97,991	9.4
Total	3,551,031	43.9	3,040,339	30.6	3,005,047	29.8	3,038,068	27.4	2,966,873	24.6

Note: Numbers are weighted to the population.
*To smooth out variation due to sampling error, average smoking rates for 10-year age groups, starting with age 25, were calculated and applied to 5-year age groups for the 1985 data.

Figure 6.1 Percentage of Canadian Population Regular Smokers by 5-Year Age Groups, Males, 1978/79–2000/01

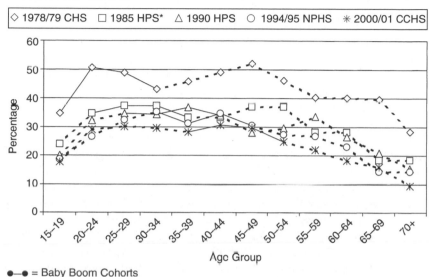

◇ 1978/79 CHS   □ 1985 HPS*   △ 1990 HPS   ○ 1994/95 NPHS   ✳ 2000/01 CCHS

●—● = Baby Boom Cohorts

Note: Each 5-year age group includes a minimum of 3 baby boom cohort years.

*To smooth out variation due to sampling error, average smoking rates for 10-year age groups, starting with age 25, were calculated and applied to 5-year age groups for the 1985 data.

2000/01, the teenage (15–19) smoking rate rises from 17.7% to 29.1% for males aged 20 to 24 and remains at about the 28% to 30% mark for subsequent years until it begins to decline rapidly around ages 50 to 54 (24.7%), dropping to a low of 9.4% for males aged 70 and over.

To examine *intra*cohort smoking trends, persons born in the same birth cohort are followed over time as they age (age effects), and then compared to other birth cohorts by reading rates diagonally in the tables. Males aged 15 to19 in 1985 exhibited a smoking rate of 23.9%. This rose to 32.2% in 1990 (aged 20–24), 32.4% in 1994/95 (about aged 25–29), and dropped back to 29.5% in 2000/01 (about aged 30–34) – point changes of +8.4%, +.2%, and –2.9%, respectively. Small *intra*cohort changes are also noted for the other age groups, including the baby boomer cohorts shown in solid lines. It can also be observed that male teenagers aged 15 to19 in 1985 experienced a more gradual rise in smoking rates over the following 15 years of their lives than the average increase based on *inter*cohort patterns. This suggests that there may be some degree of slowing in the rate of decline in smoking over time for persons born more recently compared to older cohorts.

Lower Smoking Patterns for Most Women

Turning to females, Table 6.2 and Figure 6.2 expose similar declines over the 22-year period separating the survey dates as compared with males. The bottom row in Table 6.2 (Total) shows that the percentage of the Canadian female population aged 15 and over who smoked regularly fell from 35.8% in 1978/79 to 28% in 1985, 26.8% in 1990, 23.6% in 1994/95, and 20.2% in 2000/01. As with the total male population, this dramatic drop in smoking over this period approaches half. However, when we examine period effects for specific age groups over time (comparing percentages across the same five-year age group rows of Table 6.2), it is apparent that the smoking rate for female teenagers (aged 15–19) has risen since 1990, after posting consistent and significant downswings through the late '70s and '80s. Teenage women had a smoking rate of 35.7% in 1978/79, which dropped to 21.1% in 1985, and 19% in 1990. But, it rose to 20.9% in 1994/95, which is opposite to the decline observed for all other age groups of women. Furthermore, although not shown in these tables, this incline in teenage smoking reached 25.2%, according to the 1998/99 NPHS. The rise in teenage smoking among females in the mid-1990s generated considerable targeted smoking prevention efforts. Noteworthy is that the most recent 2000/01 national data show a decline in the female teenage smoking rate to18.8%, which on a positive note is the lowest in decades. On the other hand, when we compare this 2000/01 rate of 18.8% to the 19% observed in 1990, one could argue that a decade of potential further improvement has been lost.

It is also useful to examine *inter*cohort effects by comparing female smoking rates for each five-year age group for each survey. Using the most recent 2000/01 data, it is apparent that the smoking rate for teenage women 15 to 19 (18.8%) only increases slightly throughout young adulthood, to around 25%, until ages 44 to 45, at which point it drops from 24.9% to a low of 7.7% among older women aged 70 and over. Thus, while about one in five females aged 15 to 19 smokes, we do not observe a significant increase in the smoking rates among young adult and middle-aged women. In fact, when comparisons are made across the five-year age groups for the five surveys (compare lines in Figure 6.2), it is apparent that the inverted U-shaped smoking curve that traverses the age groups is weakening for women. Moreover, we can see that the rates in 2000/01 are at their lowest point over the 22-year period under study. It is also obvious from the presentation of rates in Figure 6.2 that the

Table 6.2
Percentage of Canadian Population Regular Smokers by 5-Year Age Groups, Females, 1978/79–2000/01

| | Survey | | | | | | | | | |
| | 1978/79 CHS | | 1985 HPS* | | 1990 HPS | | 1994/95 NPHS | | 2000/01 CCHS | |
Age Group	N	%	N	%	N	%	N	%	N	%
15–19	388,450	35.7	201,848	21.1	168,40?	19.0	206,776	20.9	195,270	18.8
20–24	500,782	46.5	448,841	38.3	301,482	31.0	274,610	30.4	249,163	24.0
25–29	385,541	39.3	430,474	34.3	423,47?	35.8	346,577	32.7	218,680	22.0
30–34	310,264	36.5	331,466	34.3	412,600	34.7	377,006	27.7	233,771	22.0
35–39	288,765	42.2	321,865	31.4	364,141	33.2	368,698	29.0	330,544	25.2
40–44	223,415	37.8	231,964	31.4	273,563	27.8	284,987	25.5	335,582	24.9
45–49	233,358	41.0	182,066	30.4	198,051	25.7	247,948	26.2	282,853	23.5
50–54	202,492	35.9	198,280	30.4	189,654	29.9	159,104	21.4	222,212	21.6
55–59	182,409	34.4	158,029	24.4	151,670	25.3	126,591	18.5	150,005	19.1
60–64	110,834	26.0	130,080	24.4	122,400	20.8	137,237	22.0	105,611	16.5
65–69	81,162	22.9	128,423	17.6	89,084	16.0	78,085	13.3	82,683	13.8
70+	73,431	12.1	96,223	17.6	126,562	12.1	116,198	9.1	111,883	7.7
Total	2,980,903	35.8	2,859,559	28.0	2,821,076	25.8	2,723,817	23.6	2,518,257	20.2

Note: Numbers are weighted to the population.
*To smooth out variation due to sampling error, average smoking rates for 10-year age groups starting with age 25 were calculated and applied to 5-year age groups for the 1985 data.

Figure 6.2 Percentage of Canadian Population Regular Smokers by 5-Year Age Groups, Females, 1978/79–2000/01

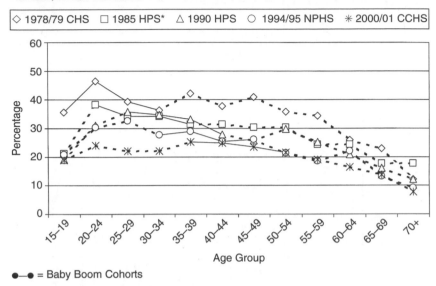

●—● = Baby Boom Cohorts

*To smooth out variation due to sampling error, average smoking rates for 10-year age groups, starting with age 25, were calculated and applied to 5-year age groups for the 1985 data.

recent decline in current smokers has been quite striking for women in their primary childbearing years, but it may be retarding for those aged 40 to 44 and above. For example, women aged 25 to 29 in 2000/01 displayed a smoking rate of only 22% compared to a remarkable 32.7% in 1994/95. Whereas, women aged 40 to 44 in 2000/01 reported a smoking rate of 24.9% compared to 25.5% in 1994/95. Thus, it would appear that an increasing number of young women are realizing the health risks of smoking, which may reflect awareness of the direct and indirect hazardous consequences of smoking for themselves as well as for their family and friends.

Investigation of *intra*cohort patterns for females reveals modest changes in aging effects on smoking, which largely mirror the ones found for males. The data suggest a reduction in the rate of decline in smoking trajectories for more recent birth cohorts over the life cycle. In sum, the period and period-cohort interactions certainly appear to be the most prominent effects in the data, which demonstrate that smoking rates have declined significantly over time for most age groups, but with opposite patterns for teenage and young women.

Gender Differences in Smoking: Dying to Be Equal

In 1978/79, there were appreciable differences in smoking rates between men and women. Overall, in 1978/79 the smoking rate for men was 8.1 percentage points higher than for women (compare bottom rows of Tables 6.1 and 6.2 for the 1978/79 column). Gender differences in smoking prevalence are also shown visually for each survey in the Appendix (Figures A1 to A5). While the rates are similar for teenage young men and women aged 15 to19 in 1978/79, adult men display higher rates for all subsequent age groups, breaking the 50% prevalence rate by their late 40s. However, these gender differences recede in the 1980s and only rise slightly in the 1990s and into 2000/01 (compare Figures A1 to A5 in Appendix). The absolute percentage gender difference is only 4.4 percentage points higher for men in 2000/01. Thus, the gendered pattern in smoking appears to be narrowing over time.

The most striking gender difference, however, is that in 2000/01, more teenage young women smoked regularly than did teenage young men – 18.8% and 17.7%, respectively. This pattern has been used to support new programmatic efforts into smoking prevention that target young women. Yet, as seen in the 2000/01 data in Figure A5, men in their 20s and 30s are smoking at considerably higher rates than females and continue to do so throughout their lives. Thus, women appear to be starting smoking earlier than men, but the rates for men catch up and surpass women's prevalence rates within just a few years. Whether the earlier timing of smoking addiction carries long-term health problems for these cohorts of women will require time to collect and assess the evidence.

How Have Exercise Patterns Changed?

In keeping with the focus on unhealthy lifestyles, the percentages of the population who are sedentary or infrequent exercisers are shown in Table 6.3 and Table 6.4. Sedentary or infrequent exercise is defined as less than three exercise intervals a week of 15 to 20 minutes or more in duration, involving vigorous activity, such as brisk walking, jogging, biking, tennis, etc. This level is considered to be below the minimum recommended level, and falls well below the level needed to gain maximum benefit from exercise. We will use the terms *unhealthy exercise*, *sedentary* or *infrequent exercise*, and *low exer-*

Table 6.3
Percentage of Canadian Population Sedentary or Infrequent Exercisers*, Males, 1978/79–2000/01

Age Group	Survey 1978/79 CHS N	%	1985 HPS N	%	1990 HPS N	%	1994/95 NPHS N	%	2000/01 CCHS N	%
15–19	316,292	28.8	207,348	20.9	233,586	24.8	231,036	24.4	215,431	22.8
20–24	463,711	44.2	466,771	38.9	313,173	31.4	291,484	37.8	334,048	35.2
25–29	497,853	53.3	438,251	41.9	609,045	51.9	442,395	44.2	361,031	39.5
30–34	493,511	59.0	484,366	42.7	673,463	57.6	503,040	42.3	418,821	42.9
35–39	417,477	61.8	472,802	46.8	583,339	54.6	665,360	52.8	495,801	43.1
40–44	336,342	61.4	379,045	50.5	557,352	57.0	469,813	44.7	529,149	43.2
45–49	381,457	68.2	299,066	50.0	479,982	62.4	472,494	50.3	471,033	44.7
50–54	352,396	67.3	380,921	57.6	298,370	47.8	383,023	51.6	395,616	42.9
55–59	317,776	66.1	372,872	60.7	322,547	54.5	280,276	49.3	304,971	42.2
60–64	245,027	67.5	219,008	46.3	282,665	52.3	230,861	45.8	211,702	38.5
65–69	193,159	61.6	230,659	50.6	210,185	45.3	191,695	38.9	171,661	35.1
70+	296,487	68.2	195,932	34.3	259,506	36.0	357,420	47.4	374,967	41.9
Total	4,311,488	55.2	4,147,041	43.6	4,823,213	48.0	4,518,897	44.2	4,284,231	39.7

Note: Numbers are weighted to the population.
*Sedentary/Infrequent exerciser = 15 min. of physical activity <3X per week.

Figure 6.3 Percentage of Canadian Population Sedentary or Infrequent Exercisers* by 5-Year Age Groups, Males, 1978/79–2000/01

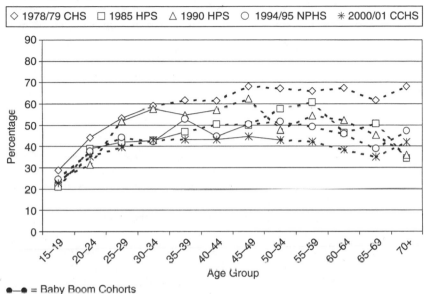

◇ 1978/79 CHS   □ 1985 HPS   △ 1990 HPS   ○ 1994/95 NPHS   ✳ 2000/01 CCHS

●—● = Baby Boom Cohorts

*15 min. of physical activity < 3X per week.

cise level interchangeably to designate this level. The data are also displayed graphically in Figures 6.3 and 6.4, and again show the baby boomer cohorts in solid.

Optimistic Exercise Patterns for Men

The bottom row of Table 6.3 shows that the percentage of males aged 15 and over who reported a sedentary or infrequent exercise level dropped markedly between 1978/79 and 2000/01, from 55.2% to 39.7%. Thus, the proportion of adult males who exercised at unhealthy levels decreased 14.9% percentage points over that period, which equals a 28% percentage drop in relative terms for this population (calculated as: 55.2% – 39.7%/55.2%). However, as seen in Figure 6.3, this decline has not been linear – the percentage of males exhibiting unhealthy physical activity levels declined significantly between 1978/79 and 1985 (55.2% to 43.6%), but actually increased to 48% in 1990. A modest drop occurred for 1994/95 (44.2%), and a similar downward trend is observed for 2000/01 to the lowest level (39.7%). Indeed, the gains made between 1978/79 and 1985 were largely lost for persons aged 15 to 49 in 1990, and it has not been until the late 1990s that we have observed significant drops in the proportion of unhealthy exercise levels beyond the 1985 rates. In other words, exercise improvements between the late 1970s and the beginning of the new millennium stalled in the late 1980s.

It can also be ascertained from Figure 6.3 that the percentage of the male population who reported being sedentary or infrequent exercisers actually peaked later across the age groups in the 1978/79 period than in 2000/01 (compare top and bottom lines of Figure 6.3). Indeed, in 1978/79, the percentage of unhealthy exercisers rose from 28.8% for persons aged 15 to 19, to 44.2% for persons aged 20 to 24, and advanced further for each five-year age group until the late 40s and early 50s, at which time the rate hovered between 60% and 70% (see first column in Table 6.3). Whereas, in 2000/01 (last percentage column in Table 6.3), the unhealthy exercise level climbed from 22.8% for the 15- to 19-year-olds, to 35.2% for those 20 to 24, and 39.5% for those 25 to 29. The rates then remain around only 40% to 45% for most of the older age groups. Thus, a different exercise trajectory across age groups has developed over time, indicating a salient period-cohort interaction effect in exercise.

Three additional major patterns can be observed by examining the individual five-year age groups. First, the decreases in the rate of unhealthy levels of exercise appear to have affected persons over the age of 30 more than those under 30. In fact, little progress has been experienced by men aged 15 to 19 over that period. Second, there are some crossover patterns among the elderly (65 to 69 and 70+) age groups. As can be seen in Figure 6.3, the significant gains in exercise observed in 1985 and 1990 appear to be lost in 1994/95 and 2000/01 for the 70+ elderly, although the most current rates are an improvement over the levels of the late 1970s. Third, middle-aged males appear to be more influenced by the reversal in unhealthy exercise around 1985 to 1990 than other age-sex cohorts.

Positive Exercise Patterns for Women

Turning to females, Table 6.4 and Figure 6.4 mirror the patterns for males over the 22-year period, except for generally higher rates of sedentary or low exercise behaviour among women in certain age groups. The bottom row in Table 6.4 tells us that the percentage of the Canadian female population aged 15 and over who exercise at levels that are defined as unhealthy decreased from 62.3% in 1978/79 to 46.7% in 1985; 50.9% in 1990; 46.8% in 1994/95; and to a low of 41% in 2000/01. This represents a 34.2% relative percentage

Table 6.4

Percentage of Canadian Population Sedentary or Infrequent Exercisers*, Females, 1978/79–2000/01

Survey

Age Group	1978/79 CHS N	%	1985 HPS N	%	1990 HPS N	%	1994/95 NPHS N	%	2000/01 CCHS N	%
15–19	378,766	35.2	264,170	27.6	291,455	32.5	338,139	36.3	308,479	32.5
20–24	569,343	54.8	495,962	42.3	474,849	48.8	336,851	39.6	340,466	35.5
25–29	592,253	62.1	495,045	45.2	619,339	52.7	513,806	49.3	348,843	37.1
30–34	548,334	65.0	518,071	46.2	671,695	56.6	625,639	47.3	401,902	39.4
35–39	450,339	67.6	487,200	53.7	640,772	58.6	626,730	49.8	515,239	40.9
40–44	365,094	66.0	442,181	52.4	561,535	57.0	519,971	48.2	545,809	41.7
45–49	379,474	69.2	284,095	49.6	416,570	54.3	434,811	47.1	468,872	40.6
50–54	384,204	69.3	305,901	44.9	303,587	47.9	375,642	51.6	396,563	40.2
55–59	326,360	64.4	285,903	51.1	275,854	45.9	257,214	38.9	315,601	41.8
60–64	290,778	72.9	313,696	50.8	268,075	45.4	249,186	41.1	238,698	39.3
65–69	267,481	76.2	231,390	43.3	244,270	43.7	260,204	46.1	234,538	41.4
70+	507,817	80.4	496,926	58.9	578,741	55.6	683,500	56.8	746,361	55.2
Total	5,060,243	62.3	4,620,540	46.7	5,346,752	50.9	5,221,693	46.8	4,861,371	41.0

Note: Numbers are weighted to the population.

*Sedentary/Infrequent exerciser = 15 min. of physical activity <3X per week.

Figure 6.4 Percentage of Canadian Population Sedentary or Infrequent Exercisers* by 5-Year Age Groups, Females, 1978/79–2000/01

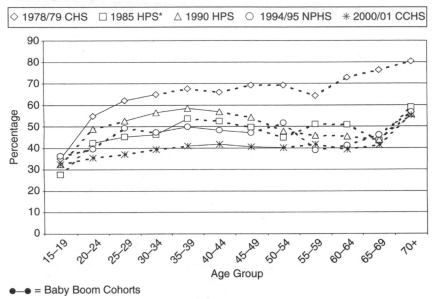

◇ 1978/79 CHS   □ 1985 HPS*   △ 1990 HPS   ○ 1994/95 NPHS   ✳ 2000/01 CCHS

●—● = Baby Boom Cohorts

*15 min. of physical activity < 3X per week.

decline in unhealthy exercise levels between 1978/79 and 2000/01 for this total population. As with males, some of the female advancements in activity levels experienced between the late 1970s and mid-1980s were lost in the late 1980s and early 1990s. In fact, almost a decade of improvement was lost between 1985 and 1994/95. However, there were substantial gains in activity patterns for both women and men over the full 22-year period under observation that is indicative of pervasive historical period effects.

Additionally, there appear to be some period-cohort interactions, since the pattern of unhealthy exercise over the full age spectrum changes shape for females as it did for males. As shown in Figure 6.4, the shape of the 2000/01 rate of unhealthy exercise is much less defined across the five-year age groups as in the past – 32.5% for women aged 15 to19, rising to 35.5% for ages 20 to 24, 37.1% for ages 25 to 29 and 39.4% for ages 30 to 34. The rate oscillates close to the 40% mark for the remaining years, except for the 70 and over age group, who exhibit an increase to 55.2%.

*Intra*cohort comparisons uncover one discernable aging pattern for females aged 15 to 19 in 1985. This cohort seems to have been more influenced by the reversal in physical activity occurring some time between 1985 and 1994/95. For most of the male and female age cohorts, the impact of this anomalous period is no more than about 10% to 12% in absolute terms. However, for females aged 15 to19, it is 21.2%. Furthermore, we do not observe that the baby boomers are the ones setting the pace for better exercise.

Gender Differences in Exercise among the Young and Old

Figures A6 to A10 (Appendix) draw on the data in Tables 6.3 and 6.4, and portray gender differences in sedentary and infrequent exercise rates separately for each survey date. This affords a clearer picture of where the sexes diverge. Generally, while the gender differences are relatively minor, there is a slight trend of higher rates of unhealthy exercise levels for teenage and older women than for their male counterparts, regardless of period or cohort. When we examine rates for specific age groups over time (comparing percentages across the rows of Table 6.4), it can be observed that unhealthy exercise rates for teenage young women (aged 15–19) have remained around 35% to 36%, except for a brief improvement shown in the 1985 survey year. While male teenagers aged 15 to 19 showed little change in their rate of unhealthy exercise, teenaged young women of this age are consistently 8 to 12 percentage points higher in sedentary or low-exercise behaviour than their male counterparts. Also, levels of unhealthy exercise are between 10 and 15 percentage points higher for elderly women than for elderly men, but mostly for the 70 and over age group. It should be noted, however, that since women outlive men, this age group may include more women who reach the upper limits of the lifespan and increased frailty, and therefore this comparison should be made with caution. On the more positive side, according to the most recent 2000/01 data, this rate does not climb appreciably, and stabilizes in the 40% range at around the same ages as for males.

Taken together, it is apparent that levels of unhealthy exercise have declined significantly for men and women between the late 1970s and the beginning of the new millennium. In the late 1970s, men aged 30 and over, and women aged 25 and over, reported unhealthy exercise levels around the 60% mark. In 2000/01, unhealthy exercise peaks around the 40% mark for the same ages. Although this is clearly an improvement (a 1/3 decline), having 40% of the population below minimum recommended levels raises concerns about Canada's population health. In addition, we have experienced a major reversal sometime between 1985 and 1994/95 with respect to exercise, and that setback influenced young women and middle-aged men the most, the latter of which includes baby boomers.

It is possible that the strong health promotion efforts targeting physical activity, such as the well-known ParticipAction program, had some degree of impact in early years but appears to have waned in the late 1980s and early 1990s. Alternatively, other historical events (i.e., recessions), or cultural shifts (i.e., changing norms) could have countered the momentum of the physical activity movement of the 1970s and early 1980s. This question will be left for a subsequent chapter to address in this book (see Chapter 12). Finally, although the genders have very similar rates of unhealthy exercise, young women and elderly women are still disadvantaged compared to men. In sum, while a majority of Canadians are active in their lifestyles, approximately 40% remain unhealthy in their levels of exercise.

How Have Patterns of Obesity Changed?

Researchers define obesity differently. A liberal definition considers persons with a body mass index (BMI) of 28 or more as obese. A more conservative definition, and one used by most Canadian researchers, as well as in the National Population Health Surveys, considers a person with a BMI of 25 to 27 as having some excess weight; a person with a BMI of 28 or above as overweight; and a person with a BMI of 30 or more to be obese. We use this definition of obesity because there is a stronger link between a BMI of 30 or more and chronic illness.

It should also be noted that the 1978/79 CHS only asked BMI information of 20% of the respondents, which resulted in unstable estimates for subgroups of the population. These data are not considered accurate enough to include in our analyses. Since BMI values are not considered to be reliable for persons less than 20 years of age and over 64, we also restrict our analyses of obesity to persons aged 20 to 64.

Obesity Patterns for Men: A Very Poor Report Card

In contrast to the declines observed in the prevalence of smoking and unhealthy exercise, an opposite picture is painted for unhealthy body weight. The overall trends between 1985 and 2000/01, a period of approximately 16 years, show more than a *doubling* of the prevalence of obesity among adult Canadian males ages 20 to 64. The rate has increased rapidly, from an estimated 7.1% in 1985 to 10.5% in 1990, 14% in 1994/95, and a striking 16.3% in 2000/01 (see bottom row, Table 6.5). This inflation in obesity is alarming given the relatively short interval under study. It is also consistent with many other North American studies documenting this trend, as covered in Chapter 4. The rise in

Table 6.5
Percentage of Canadian Population Obese (BMI = 30+) by 5-Year Age Groups, Males, 1985–2000/01*

| | Survey | | | | | | | |
| | 1985 HPS* | | 1990 HPS | | 1994/95 NPHS | | 2000/01 CCHS | |
Age Group	N	%	N	%	N	%	N	%
20–24	32,325	2.7	35,173	3.5	69,162	8.3	85,147	8.0
25–29	36,998	3.5	70,926	6.1	130,656	12.2	145,987	14.5
30–34	40,811	3.6	107,887	9.2	130,696	10.4	168,112	15.5
35–39	84,162	8.3	99,678	9.3	156,351	11.9	204,791	16.2
40–44	38,704	5.1	118,550	12.1	158,101	13.8	225,190	16.7
45–49	81,612	13.6	73,667	9.6	162,940	16.2	219,709	18.9
50–54	63,804	10.0	116,116	18.7	154,083	19.4	216,441	21.3
55–59	47,366	7.7	83,455	14.3	88,810	15.0	154,831	19.5
60–64	45,916	9.4	64,583	11.8	103,948	18.9	106,422	17.7
Total	471,698	7.1	770,035	10.5	1,154,747	14.0	1,526,630	16.3

Note: BMI values are not reliable for persons under age 20 and over age 64, and therefore are not included. Numbers are weighted to the population.
*Since BMI was collected only for a sub-sample composed of about 20% of the 1978/79 CHS sample, the population estimates are unreliable and have been omitted.

Figure 6.5 Percentage of Canadian Population Obese (BMI 30+) by 5-Year Age Groups, Males, 1985–2000/01

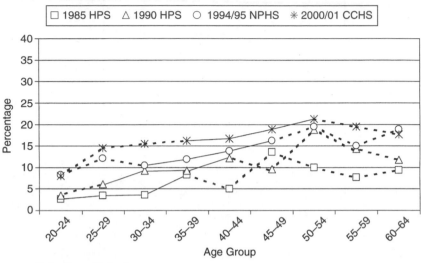

●—● = Baby Boom Cohorts

Note: Since BMI was collected for only a 20% sub-sample of the 1978/79 CHS, the population estimates are unreliable and have been omitted.

obesity has been consistent over these years, exhibiting an almost perfect linear increase in the overall population rates between the mid-1980s and the early years of the new millennium. It will also be seen that this pattern cannot be blamed on the baby boomers, but rather reflects a fundamental shift in population health.

Interestingly, the period patterns shown for males by five-year age groups are quite diverse, but confirm a general increase in obesity. This can be seen by examining the individual row percentages in Table 6.5 and by comparing the four survey points for each age group. It can also be visually observed in Figure 6.5. While there is an upward trajectory in obesity over time, the rate for men in their 20s appears to be slowing in recent years. Conversely, the rate has risen faster for men in their middle years. For example, men aged 40 to 44 have reported prevalence rates in obesity from 5.1% in 1985, to 12.1% in 1990, 13.8% in 1994/95, and 16.7% in 2000/01. This is a more than *tripling* of the rate, much of which appears to have occurred between the mid-'80s and the early 1990s, and therefore includes the younger baby boomers in this period-cohort interaction. It is also noteworthy that this occurred during the same historical period in which unhealthy exercise levels exhibited a temporary reversal.

Comparing the column percentages for each survey date identifies *inter*cohort effects and their interactions. Overall, male obesity tends to rise fairly consistently by age for any particular survey year, rising throughout the young adult and midlife years, peaking in the early 50s, and showing gradual declines thereafter to age 64. It is also apparent from these data that there is a steeper slope to this incline since the 1990s, such that male obesity rates reach the 10% and higher threshold by the time males reach their mid-20s, whereas in 1985 they did not hit this watermark until they were in their late 40s. Specifically, in 2000/01 the male prevalence of obesity moves from 8% for males aged 20 to 24 to 14.5% for males 25 to 29, whereas back in 1985 the male obesity rate starts at only 2.7% for the 20 to 24 age group, increases more gradually to 8.3% for males aged 35 to 39, and peaks at only 13.6% for the 45- to 49-year-olds. Figure 6.5 depicts these period-cohort patterns graphically, and underscores the seriousness of this dramatic trend in unhealthy body mass.

Comparative analyses of the data indicate that for both men and women, there are relatively minor pure aging effects over time, and, moreover, that it appears that the most important shifts relate to age, period, and cohort interactions. Two noteworthy patterns are (1) steeper inclines in obesity rates when people are in their 20s, and (2) a consistent rise in obesity over the time period between 1985 and 2000/01.

Obesity Patterns for Women: Another Poor Report Card

The obesity epidemic is as serious for women as it is for men. Between 1985 and 2000/01 there has been more than a *doubling* of the prevalence of obesity among adult Canadian females aged 20 to 64 (see bottom row, Table 6.6). The rate has increased from an estimated 5.8% in 1985, to 9.7% in 1990, 14% in 1994/95, and 14.2% in 2000/01. As it is for males, this rise in the female obesity rate is astounding, given that it has occurred over such a short period, and the fact that it shows a consistent upward trajectory.

Again, the period trends for the five-year age group reveal some diversity, but overall reflect growing body mass between 1985 and 2000/01. This is observed by examining the row percentages in Table 6.6 and by comparing the four survey points for each five-year age group in Figure 6.6. The most rapid incline in obesity rate over this time period appears to be for women in their late 20s and for those aged 50 and over. For example, between 1985 and 2000/01, women aged 25 to 29 experienced a six-fold rise in obesity rate, from 1.8% to 11.2%, and those aged 55 to 59 experienced a four-fold increase, from 5.1%

Table 6.6
Percentage of Canadian Population Obese (BMI = 30+) by 5-Year Age Groups, Females, 1985–2000/01*

Age Group	Survey							
	1985 HPS*		1990 HPS		1994/95 NPHS		2000/01 CCHS	
	N	%	N	%	N	%	N	%
20–24	15,430	1.3	23,535	2.4	75,929	8.9	72,485	7.4
25–29	19,788	1.8	52,334	4.5	116,134	12.4	100,643	11.2
30–34	41,398	3.7	98,508	8.3	139,775	10.9	121,075	12.4
35–39	57,994	6.5	80,399	7.5	153,746	12.6	170,599	13.6
40–44	67,824	8.2	116,791	12.0	141,552	13.0	179,128	13.8
45–49	46,898	8.4	84,058	11.0	152,291	16.7	180,620	15.5
50–54	52,199	7.8	68,969	11.0	103,240	14.0	178,418	17.9
55–59	28,435	5.1	96,224	16.1	110,023	16.3	152,933	20.2
60–64	60,742	9.7	83,609	14.4	128,506	20.8	117,066	18.7
Total	390,708	5.8	704,427	9.7	1,121,196	14.0	1,272,967	14.2

Note: BMI values are not reliable for persons under age 20 and over age 64, and therefore are not included. Numbers are weighted to the population.
*Since BMI was collected only for a sub-sample composed of about 20% of the 1978/79 CHS sample, the population estimates are unreliable and have been omitted.

Figure 6.6 Percentage of Canadian Population Obese (BMI 30+) by 5-Year Age Groups, Females, 1985–2000/01

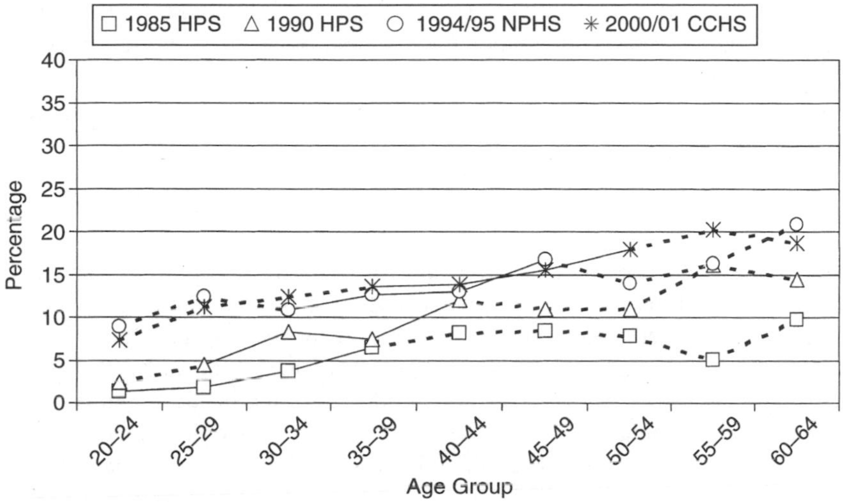

●—● = Baby Boom Cohorts

Note: Since BMI was collected for only a 20% sub-sample of the 1978/79 CHS, the population estimates are unreliable and have been omitted.

to 20.2%. There is a glimmer of hope, however, in that the 2000/01 rate has dropped slightly below the 1994/95 rate for females in their 20s, as well as those aged 40 to 49 and 60 to 64. This may be indicative of either a reversal in this trend or at least a threshold in obesity being reached among Canadian females.

*Inter*cohort patterns reveal that female obesity tends to be highest among women in their late 40s and late 50s, with a slight drop among those aged 60 to 64. Comparing survey dates, it can also be clearly seen that that the slope of the incline for females in their 20s has been much steeper in 2000/01 than it was in earlier years. Examining the column percentages for 2000/01, for example, the obesity rate jumps from 7.4% among women aged 20 to 24, to 11.2% among those aged 25 to 29, already crossing the 10% watermark. In 1985, the comparable rates were only 1.3% for women aged 20 to 24, and only 1.8% for aged 25 to 29.

Gender Differences in Obesity: Equality of the Worst Kind

Figures A11 to A14 (see Appendix) exhibit gender differences in obesity for each survey year separately drawn from the data presented in Tables 6.5 and

6.6. Two findings are particularly dominant. First, obesity rates for men are slightly worse than for women because of higher obesity rates in the middle years of life – 40s and 50s. Second, the obesity rates for young adults in their 20s and 30s are extremely similar for men and women, except for 2000/01, where it can be seen that men display slightly higher rates across all ages. The one exception is that, after age 55 to 59, women outweigh men proportionate to height.

Average Body Mass Index Patterns: A Population Health Problem

The average BMI for males and females is mapped in Figures 6.7 and 6.8, drawing from Tables 6.7 and 6.8, respectively. These presentations are useful because they reflect the broader shifts in BMI for the total population rather than using an arbitrary cut-off point (i.e., BMI 30+), and therefore help to elucidate key trends. These tables and graphs confirm a steady rise in BMI for the Canadian population between 1985 and 2000/01, one that has pushed us past important thresholds. They demonstrate that over that same period, we

Figure 6.7 Mean Body Mass Index (BMI) of Canadian Population by 5-Year Age Groups, Males, 1985–2000/0

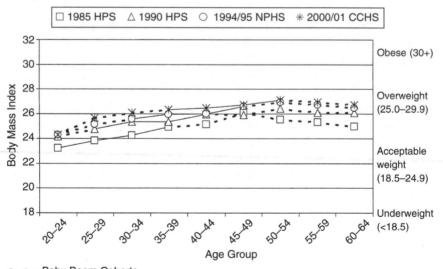

●—● = Baby Boom Cohorts

Note: Since BMI was collected for only a 20% sub-sample of the 1978/79 CHS, the population estimates are unreliable and have been omitted.

Table 6.7
Mean BMI of the Canadian Population, Males, 1985–2000/01*

Age Group	Survey			
	1985 HPS	1990 HPS	1994/95 NPHS	2000/01 CCHS
20–24	23.23	24.18	24.31	24.31
25–29	23.82	24.78	25.15	25.67
30–34	24.27	25.38	25.58	26.10
35–39	24.94	25.36	25.97	26.36
40–44	25.16	25.96	26.01	26.46
45–49	26.10	25.92	26.60	26.75
50–54	25.51	26.43	26.93	27.10
55–59	25.31	26.08	26.75	26.93
60–64	24.99	26.10	26.48	26.73
Total	24.81	25.58	25.98	26.24

Note: BMI values are not reliable for persons under age 20 and over age 64 and therefore are not included.
*Since BMI was collected only for a sub-sample composed of about 20% of the 1978/79 CHS sample, the population estimates are unreliable and have been omitted.

Table 6.8
Mean BMI of the Canadian Population, Females, 1985–2000/01*

Age Group	Survey			
	1985 HPS	1990 HPS	1994/95 NPHS	2000/01 CCHS
20–24	21.39	21.89	23.05	22.79
25–29	22.03	22.32	23.68	23.89
30–34	22.20	23.20	23.92	24.36
35–39	22.86	24.43	23.98	24.49
40–44	23.67	24.44	24.70	24.78
45–49	23.83	24.50	25.45	25.40
50–54	24.40	24.41	25.63	26.01
55–59	24.69	25.17	26.05	26.27
60–64	24.60	25.23	26.04	26.20
Total	23.30	23.95	24.72	24.83

Note: BMI values are not reliable for persons under age 20 and over age 64 and therefore are not included.
*Since BMI was collected only for a sub-sample composed of about 20% of the 1978/79 CHS sample, the population estimates are unreliable and have been omitted.

Figure 6.8 Mean Body Mass Index (BMI) of Canadian Population by 5-Year Age Groups, Females, 1985–2000/0

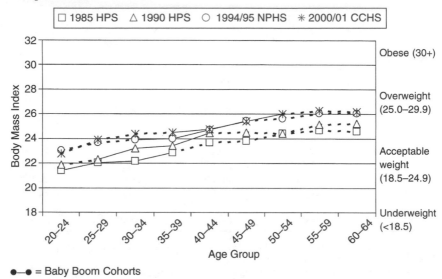

●—● = Baby Boom Cohorts

Note: Since BMI was collected for only a 20% sub-sample of the 1978/79 CHS, the population estimates are unreliable and have been omitted.

have moved from an adult population exhibiting an average BMI in the acceptable weight range (defined as BMI 18.5 to 24.9) to one that has moved into the overweight level (defined as BMI 25 to 29.9). For the male population aged 20 to 64, the average BMI increased from 24.81 in 1985 to 26.24 in 2000/01, and from 23.30 to 24.83 for females. It is also clear from the five-year age data in Tables 6.7 and 6.8, that in 2000/01, the crossing of the overweight threshold (BMI 25+) occurred earlier in the lives of men and women. The 25 and over BMI level was reached among males in their late 20s and among females in their late 40s in 2000/01, whereas, in 1985 this occurred among males in their early 40s, and women never reached this threshold.

How Have Patterns of Heavy Drinking Changed?

The fourth unhealthy behaviour to be examined is heavy drinking. This is defined as 14 or more drinks per week for men and 12 or more for women, given their lower body weight. The percentages of the population who are heavy drinkers by five-year age group are shown in Table 6.9 and Table 6.10.

As previously discussed, this level is considered to place individuals at risk for a number of major health conditions, and will be deemed unhealthy.

Patterns of Heavy Drinking for Men: The Good and the Bad

The bottom row of Table 6.9 (see p. 90) shows that the percentage of males aged 15 and over who reported heavy drinking fell dramatically between 1978/79 and 2000/01, from 21.8% in 1978/79 to 13.1% in 1985, 13.2% in 1990, 9.9% in 1994/95, and 10.1% in 2000/01. Thus, the proportion of the adult male population who drink at unhealthy levels has decreased by *more than half* over that time period. Even taking into account that a 6.5-year period separates the first two surveys, it can be seen that the largest drop in heavy drinking occurred between 1978/79 and 1985 (also see Figure 6.9). Thus, these data signify that the late 1970s represent the tail end of a period in history when a high level of drinking was considered to be acceptable in society, as depicted on television and the movies.

The reduction in rates of heavy drinking among males has been particularly striking for certain age groups. Rates of heavy drinking have shown significant but modest decreases for teenage males aged 15 to 19 between 1978/79 and 1994/95, and, furthermore, some of this improvement appears to be lost between the mid-1990s and early 2000s (see Table 6.9 and Figure 6.9). However, a much larger drop has occurred among young men. For example, the prevalence of heavy drinking among males aged 20 to 24 shrunk from 32.4% in 1978/79 to only 11.9% in 1994/95, but has since risen slightly, to 15.3% in 2000/01. This pattern is replicated for most adult ages (compare patterns in Figure 6.9).

Also apparent from these data is that there is a smoothing of the pattern of heavy drinking across age groups over time. In 1978/79 and 1985, in particular, the rates of heavy drinking have severe gradients, especially at the younger and older ages, whereas in 2000/01 the changes are more modest, and, indeed, the prevalence of heavy drinking in 2000/01 oscillates around the 10% level for all age groups until the age of 70. The one exception is for teenage and young adults. In 2000/01, these groups exhibit an incline in the prevalence of heavy drinking, from 7.2% (ages 15 to 19) to 15.3% (ages 20 to 24), followed by a drop to 13.1% (ages 25 to 29). Thus, health promotion efforts and shifts in normative expectations seem to have reduced the prevalence of heavy drinking, especially in the male population between 1978/79 and 2000/01. However, there appears to be a slowdown, and, indeed, a small reversal in this trend for several age groups in the late 1990s, especially among teenagers and young adults. The *intra*cohort patterns of heavy drinking for males and females indicate relatively small aging effects compared to period and cohort effects.

Table 6.9
Percentage of Canadian Population Heavy Drinkers* by 5-Year Age Groups, Males, 1978/79–2000/01

| | Survey | | | | | | | | | |
| | 1978/79 CHS | | 1985 HPS**° | | 1990 HPS | | 1994/95 NPHS | | 2000/01 CCHS | |
Age Group	N	%	N	%	N	%	N	%	N	%
15–19	149,350	14.4	94,000	9.5	131,528	14.0	65,848	6.2	77,685	7.2
20–24	343,283	32.4	214,038	17.9	202,294	20.3	99,037	11.9	159,673	15.3
25–29	255,377	27.5	130,622	12.9	195,451	16.7	138,152	12.8	130,979	13.1
30–34	186,936	22.5	154,542	12.9	160,326	13.7	130,359	10.4	104,266	9.6
35–39	143,266	21.7	126,945	17.8	130,234	12.1	124,553	9.5	107,253	8.5
40–44	114,616	20.9	170,203	17.8	116,893	12.0	120,083	10.5	120,970	9.0
45–49	121,589	22.1	39,644	11.8	108,845	14.1	113,777	11.3	115,218	10.0
50–54	107,201	20.8	111,745	11.8	74,803	12.1	64,733	8.2	109,979	10.9
55–59	95,724	21.3	73,753	12.7	57,663	9.9	44,986	7.6	85,114	10.7
60–64	65,588	18.0	64,952	12.7	48,057	8.8	78,906	14.4	55,323	9.2
65–69	46,722	16.0	42,283	9.7	53,062	11.5	48,692	9.4	60,013	11.0
70+	41,383	9.8	58,783	9.7	40,652	5.6	54,883	6.3	75,758	7.3
Total	1,671,035	21.8	1,281,510	13.1	1,319,808	13.2	1,084,009	9.9	1,202,231	10.1

Note: Numbers are weighted to the population.
*Heavy drinker = 14+ drinks/week for males and 12+ drinks/week for females.
**The midpoint of categories representing a range of number of drinks consumed per week was used as an estimate of drinking behaviour for the 1985 HPS data; since the highest category was 12+ drinks, these calculations may underestimate the percentage of heavy drinkers for this year.
°To smooth out variation due to sampling error, average rates of heavy drinking for 10-year age groups, starting with age 25, were calculated and applied to 5-year age groups for the 1985 data.

Table 6.10

Percentage of Canadian Population Heavy Drinkers* by 5-Year Age Groups, Females, 1978/79–2000/01

| | Survey | | | | | | | | | |
| | 1978/79 CHS | | 1985 HPS***° | | 1990 HPS | | 1994/95 NPHS | | 2000/01 CCHS | |
Age Group	N	%	N	%	N	%	N	%	N	%
15–19	77,265	7.4	31,856	3.3	32,363	3.7	26,206	2.7	36,249	3.5
20–24	110,506	10.4	61,911	5.3	38,997	4.1	38,878	4.3	53,976	5.2
25–29	71,583	7.5	49,379	3.6	31,841	2.7	30,815	2.9	31,544	3.2
30–34	57,215	6.8	28,514	3.6	35,058	3.0	36,236	2.7	24,743	2.3
35–39	63,716	9.7	11,529	2.5	29,920	2.7	40,023	3.2	41,971	3.2
40–44	30,336	5.4	31,368	2.5	24,627	2.5	34,430	3.1	49,260	3.7
45–49	30,939	5.8	28,031	4.3	22,207	2.9	29,380	3.1	41,755	3.5
50–54	35,647	6.6	25,042	4.3	26,936	4.3	17,374	2.3	22,725	2.2
55–59	42,043	8.7	23,007	3.8	16,654	2.8	13,961	2.1	21,727	2.8
60–64	14,858	3.9	20,537	3.8	13,141	2.2	18,102	2.9	19,655	3.1
65–69	12,443	3.7	9,307	1.5	14,529	2.6	13,703	2.4	15,997	2.7
70+	10,849	1.9	10,398	1.5	23,472	2.3	27,182	2.1	27,915	1.9
Total	557,400	7.0	330,879	3.3	309,739	3.0	326,290	2.8	387,517	3.1

Note: Numbers are weighted to the population.

*Heavy drinker = 14+ drinks/week for males and 12+ drinks/week for females.

**The midpoint of categories representing a range of numbers of drinks consumed per week was used as an estimate of drinking behaviour for the 1985 HPS data; since the highest category was 12+ drinks, these calculations may underestimate the percentage of heavy drinkers for this year.

°To smooth out variation due to sampling error, average rates of heavy drinking for 10-year age groups, starting with age 25, were calculated and applied to 5-year age groups for the 1985 data.

Figure 6.9 Percentage of Canadian Population Heavy Drinkers* by 5-Year Age Groups, Males, 1978/79–2000/01

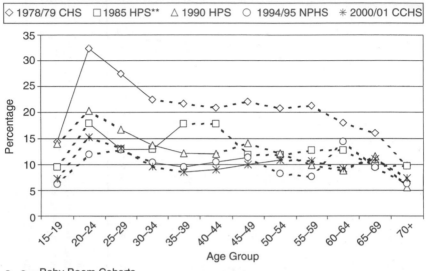

●—● = Baby Boom Cohorts

*14+ drinks/week.
**To smooth out variation due to sampling error, average smoking rates for 10-year age groups, starting with age 25, were calculated and applied to 5-year age groups for the 1985 data.

Patterns of Heavy Drinking for Women: The Age Factor

Table 6.10 and Figure 6.10 present the prevalence rates for heavy drinking for women. The general patterns observed are very similar for women and for men, except that the rates are considerably lower for women (see subsequent section). The bottom row of Table 6.10 demonstrates a downturn in the percentage of females aged 15 and over who reported heavy drinking – from 7% in 1978/79 to 3.3% in 1985, 3% in 1990, 2.8% in 1994/95, and 3.1% in 2000/01. Thus, the rate of heavy drinking among women has also dropped by *more than half* over this time period. The largest decrease in the rate of heavy drinking among females between 1978/79 and 2000/01 appear to have been among those aged 15 to 39, and among those in their 50s (examine row percentages in Table 6.10). Smaller improvements can be seen for women in their 40s.

Figure 6.10 Percentage of Canadian Population Heavy Drinkers* by 5-Year Age Groups, Females, 1978/79–2000/01

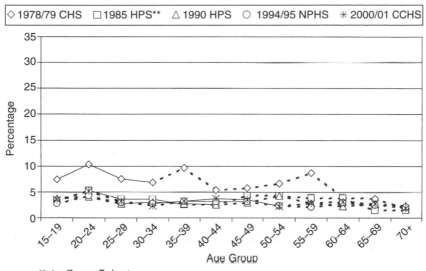

●—● = Baby Boom Cohorts

*12+ drinks/week.
**To smooth out variation due to sampling error, average smoking rates for 10-year age groups, starting with age 25, were calculated and applied to 5-year age groups for the 1985 data.

As with the male patterns, it can also be observed from Figure 6.10 that there seems to be a softening of the age pattern of heavy drinking over time for women. In particular, in 1978/79, the rate zigzags considerably across the age groups. However, in 2000/01, the changes are slight and the rate of heavy drinking hovers around only 2% to 4%. Overall, the prevalence of heavy drinking in the female population has continued to drop during this period, even among teenagers. But, as with males, there are indications of a slow-down, and even a small reversal, in this trend in the late 1990s and early 2000s.

Gender Differences in Heavy Drinking: It's Worse Than You Think

Tables 6.9 and 6.10 can also be used to highlight gender differences in heavy drinking for each survey date. Figures A15 to A19 (Appendix) have been constructed from these data to reflect these patterns. As observed in these data, there are enormous gender differences in heavy drinking, which is more of a male than a female health issue. However, if one examines the extent of the gender differences for each successive survey, it becomes apparent that the gender gap in heavy drinking has been narrowing over time. The greatest drop has occurred for men in their 20s between 1978/79 and 1985, and is probably the consequence of the very high male rates in these ages falling faster than the lower female rates of heavy drinking. Still, male patterns in 2000/01 have not reached the 1978/79 female levels. And, furthermore, while the 2000/01 female rate in heavy drinking fluctuates between about 3% and 5% across the ages forming the life cycle, the rate for men oscillates between about 10% and 15%, except among teenagers and elderly men aged 70 and over, who have rates of heavy drinking near 7%. Overall, while gender differences in heavy drinking have shown significant declines over this time period, men continue to drink at unhealthy levels at approximately *three times* the female rate. Baby boomers generally mirror these patterns, and will be given special attention in Chapter 8.

7

Population Changes in Health Status and Health Utilization

This chapter examines period changes in four measures of chronic illness (total chronic conditions, hypertension, arthritis, and diabetes), as well as doctor visits. Measures of chronic illness were not collected in the 1985 and 1990 HPS. Since these measures are only available in surveys that are not evenly spaced over a significant period of time – the 1978/79 CHS, 1994/95 NPHS, 1998/99NPHS, and 2000/01 CCHS – a full age-period-cohort analysis is not possible. Only period trends are presented to show changes in rates over time. Male and female rates are discussed separately. Two types of comparisons of rates are made: (1) absolute percentage differences (calculated by subtracting one percentage from another); and (2) relative percentage change (calculated by subtracting one rate from a second rate, and dividing by the first rate). Since the individual chronic illnesses occur at very small rates among younger age groups (e.g., hypertension), we begin with either the 40 to 44 or 45 to 49 five-year age groups. This places obvious limitations on an age-period-cohort analysis of persons in the baby boomer cohorts in this section. Chapter 8 specifically addresses baby boomer health dynamics using a different method. Furthermore, analyses of prescription medications proved to be problematic and had to be omitted, since its measurement changed significantly over the surveys, and the 2000/01 survey only collected this information from persons living in Ontario.

The data presented in this chapter need to be interpreted with some degree of caution because of several limitations. It should be noted that these data are based on self-reports. Also, shifts over time in health status information may reflect changes in detection of illness rather than actual changes in prevalence rates over time, since they are based on an individual's perception of being diagnosed by a medical professional.

Table 7.1
Percentage of Canadian Population with a Chronic Condition by 5-Year Age Groups, Males, 1978/79–2000/01*

| | Survey | | | | | | | |
| | 1978/79 CHS | | 1994/95 NPHS | | 1998/99 NPHS | | 2000/01 CCHS | |
Age Group	N	%	N	%	N	%	N	%
15–19	313,162	26.4	441,911	41.8	489,276	44.9	481,467	44.2
20–24	367,861	33.2	312,327	37.3	387,727	40.0	472,488	44.2
25–29	375,912	38.0	414,394	38.3	433,813	46.5	488,730	48.5
30–34	323,748	35.8	567,319	45.2	553,200	50.4	531,479	49.1
35–39	289,288	40.4	581,466	44.0	605,350	44.5	691,936	54.6
40–44	248,684	40.2	556,147	48.3	739,549	53.7	751,721	55.8
45–49	326,469	52.3	521,814	51.1	549,891	54.6	689,012	59.5
50–54	354,751	60.1	471,723	59.2	553,974	58.9	641,691	63.3
55–59	330,601	62.1	388,470	64.6	464,170	64.2	561,631	70.6
60–64	309,165	72.2	379,440	68.9	443,823	71.0	465,397	78.0
65–69	275,511	77.2	385,433	73.6	379,745	76.9	428,631	78.9
70+	420,553	79.4	693,987	79.3	851,487	84.1	886,979	86.2
Total	3,935,705	45.8	5,714,431	51.6	6,452,005	55.5	7,091,162	59.1

Note: Numbers are weighted to the population.
*1985 and 1990 data are not available for chronic conditions.

Figure 7.1 Percentage of Canadian Population with a Chronic Condition by 5-Year Age Groups, Males, 1978/79–2000/01

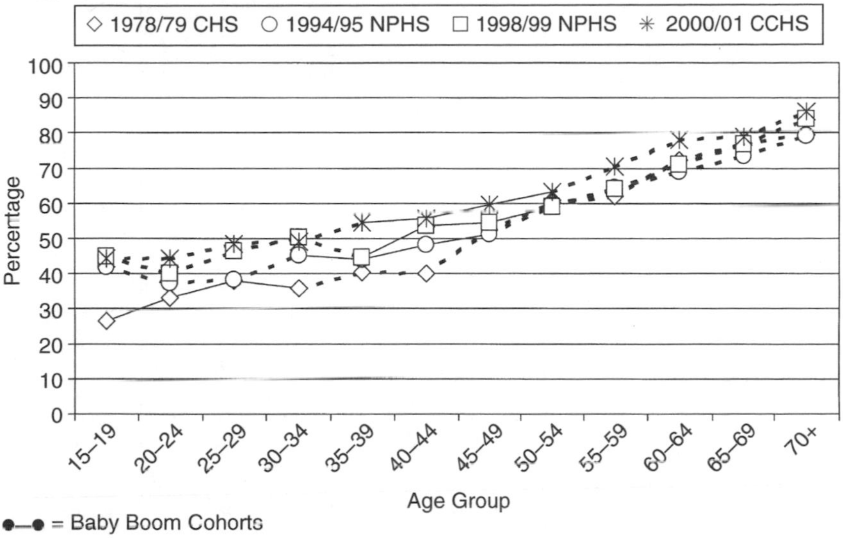

●—● = Baby Boom Cohorts

Note: 1985 and 1990 data are not available for chronic conditions.

Trends in Chronic Illness for Males: A Recent Upturn

The first health measure displays the percentage of persons reporting any chronic illness. This broad measure includes a wide range of illnesses, including asthma, arthritis, diabetes, hypertension, heart problems, and so on. There has been a pattern of increasing prevalence of chronic conditions among males between 1978/79 and 2000/01, as shown in Table 7.1. For all age groups (bottom row), the rate of chronic illness has inflated modestly (about 15%), from 45.8% in 1978/79 to 51.6% in 1994/95, 55.5% in 1998/99, and 59.1% in 2000/01. As can be seen in Table 7.1 and visually presented in Figure 7.1, most of this increase over the years in question has actually occurred among persons under age 50 during this period, rather than among older adults. However, a more pronounced aging pattern observed in these data is that, for all four time periods, rates of chronic conditions rise sharply after age 50, from about 50% of the male population at age 50 to 54 to approximately 80% for persons aged 70 and over.

Higher Levels and Increases in Chronic Illness for Females

Table 7.2 and Figure 7.2 reflect a very similar pattern for females as for males – there is a marked incline in the prevalence of chronic illness across the

Table 7.2
Percentage of Canadian Population with a Chronic Condition by 5-Year Age Groups, Females, 1978/79–2000/01*

| | Survey | | | | | | | |
| | 1978/79 CHS | | 1994/95 NPHS | | 1998/99 NPHS | | 2000/01 CCHS | |
Age Group	N	%	N	%	N	%	N	%
15–19	385,484	33.6	458,981	46.4	485,812	46.4	548,720	53.0
20–24	471,633	42.6	411,218	45.6	519,467	54.2	607,862	58.8
25–29	450,239	44.8	528,126	49.9	483,378	55.4	611,380	61.7
30–34	401,812	44.4	678,504	49.9	667,308	55.2	658,362	62.0
35–39	338,366	47.4	615,027	48.3	831,843	59.6	829,263	63.6
40–44	365,275	59.3	583,215	52.2	769,451	60.0	885,572	66.1
45–49	371,538	60.2	546,044	57.8	759,303	68.8	832,001	69.5
50–54	413,025	67.6	459,869	62.0	666,565	72.5	771,864	75.4
55–59	426,297	73.8	489,900	71.6	493,275	77.0	611,865	79.0
60–64	384,239	81.2	435,729	69.7	556,809	80.8	532,655	83.8
65–69	322,084	79.3	451,358	77.6	501,600	83.2	502,211	84.3
70+	618,266	85.1	1,087,424	85.6	1,196,196	88.6	1,306,490	91.4
Total	4,948,258	55.6	6,745,395	58.4	7,931,007	65.7	8,698,245	70.0

Note: Numbers are weighted to the population.
*1985 and 1990 data are not available for chronic conditions.

Figure 7.2 Percentage of Canadian Population with a Chronic Condition by 5-Year Age Groups, Females, 1978/79–2000/01

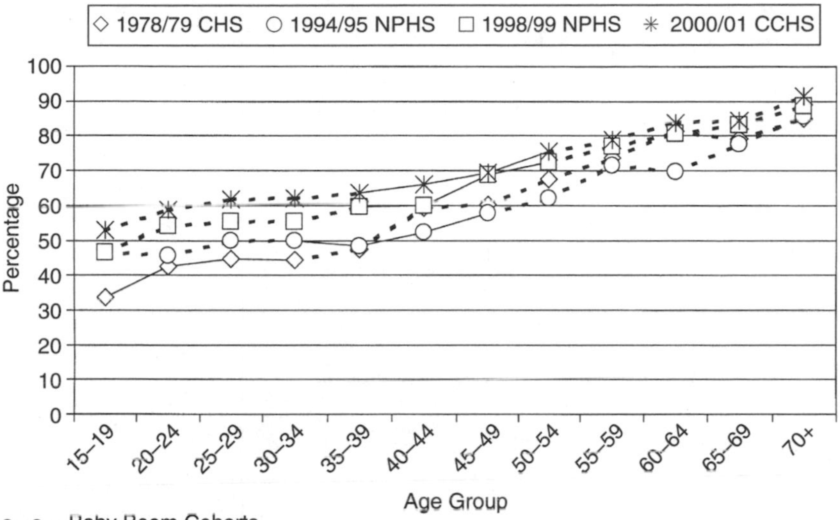

◇ 1978/79 CHS   ○ 1994/95 NPHS   □ 1998/99 NPHS   ✳ 2000/01 CCHS

●—● = Baby Boom Cohorts

Note: 1985 and 1990 data are not available for chronic conditions.

survey dates, and there appears to be a larger increase for women under 50 than over 50. Also noteworthy is that the rates of chronic illness are higher for women than for men by about 10% (10 percentage points) at virtually every age. Thus, we see a rise from 55.6% in 1978/79 to 58.4% in 1994/95, 65.7% in 1998/99, and 70% in 2000/01 (see bottom row of Table 7.2). As can be seen in these data, the prevalence of chronic illness appears to have shifted upward the greatest since 1994/95. In addition, it is portentous that teenage females aged 15 to 19 (as well as males) have experienced about a 20 percentage point rise in the prevalence of chronic illness, or about a 60% relative increase. The pattern of chronic illness across the ages comprising the life cycle of females also depicts an upward linear pattern with age, similar to males. Again, the fact that diagnostic procedures have become more sensitive over this time period may account for some of the inflation in rates of chronic illness.

Rising Rates of Hypertension for Men

Hypertension is a major risk factor for cardiovascular disease and diabetes. Tables 7.3 and 7.4 present hypertension rates for males and females who are aged 45 and over. This higher-age starting point is selected because of the

Table 7.3 Percentage of Canadian Population with Hypertension, Males 45+, 1978/79–2000/01*

Age Group	Survey							
	1978/79 CHS		1994/95 NPHS		1998/99 NPHS		2000/01 CCHS	
	N	%	N	%	N	%	N	%
45–49	51,144	8.2	68,493	6.7	78,062	7.8	134,217	11.5
50–54	86,938	14.7	104,690	13.2	119,822	12.7	164,073	16.1
55–59	49,977	9.4	109,078	18.2	142,911	19.8	173,585	21.7
60–64	80,460	18.8	102,442	18.6	153,469	24.4	167,607	27.8
65–69	67,549	18.9	128,638	24.6	135,558	27.5	176,336	32.2
70+	107,024	20.2	198,870	22.8	306,869	30.1	362,325	34.8
Total	443,092	15.0	712,211	17.4	936,691	20.4	1,178,143	24.0

Note: Numbers are weighted to the population.
*1985 and 1990 data are not available for chronic conditions.

Figure 7.3 Percentage of Canadian Population with Hypertension by 5-Year Age Groups, Males, 1978/79–2000/01

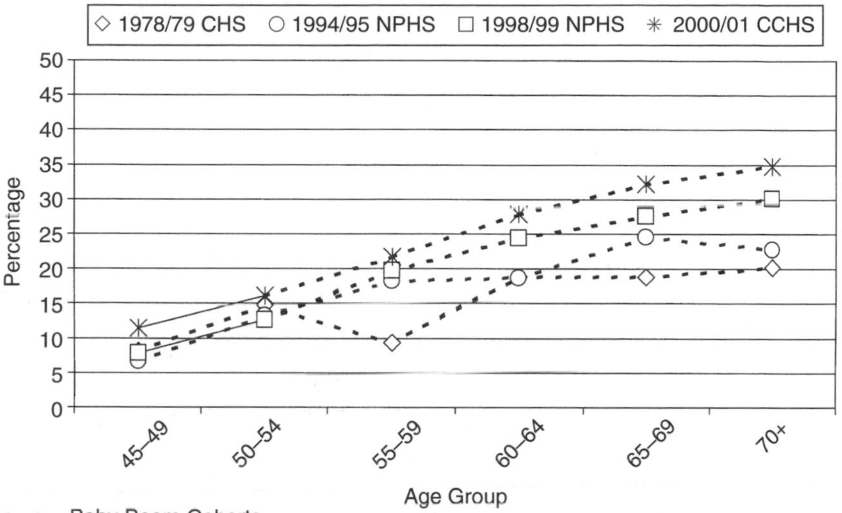

●—● = Baby Boom Cohorts

Note: 1985 and 1990 data are not available for chronic conditions.

extremely low rates among persons under that age, which makes estimation procedures tenuous. It should be recalled also that confidence intervals have been calculated for hypertension and all other individual chronic illnesses because the rates of single illnesses are based on distributions that are prone to sampling variability. Since the confidence intervals are still relatively small – less than plus or minus 2% – only the calculated rates are shown in the tables. However, the confidence intervals are used to assess changes in the prevalence rates – that is, shifts in rates that are smaller than the confidence interval are concluded to be due potentially to sampling error. Similar to the prevalence of chronic illness, the hypertension rate for males exhibits a slow but steady rise that has been gaining momentum over the last decade. The hypertension rate for males aged 45 and over is 15% in 1978/79, 17.4% in 1994/95, 20.4% in 1998/99, and 24% in 2000/01. The relative percentage increase in hypertension between 1978/79 and 1994/95 is 16%; however, between 1994/95 and 2000/01 (only six years) it is approximately 38%.

Another prominent trend is the insidious incline in hypertension rates with older age groups, regardless of survey date (see Figure 7.3). Taking 2000/01 as an example, the prevalence rate of high blood pressure for males rose in a

Table 7.4
Percentage of Canadian Population with Hypertension, Females 45+, 1978/79–2000/01*

Age Group	Survey							
	1978/79 CHS		1994/95 NPHS		1998/99 NPHS		2000/01 CCHS	
	N	%	N	%	N	%	N	%
45–49	62,479	10.1	80,391	8.5	84,347	7.6	136,327	11.3
50–54	108,366	17.7	97,296	13.1	159,337	17.3	192,552	18.7
55–59	130,359	22.6	139,249	20.4	134,704	20.8	199,013	25.4
60–64	134,964	28.5	155,147	24.9	220,414	31.9	195,611	30.6
65–69	125,002	30.8	169,706	29.2	242,258	40.1	220,039	36.6
70+	273,076	37.6	432,643	34.1	585,448	42.9	648,920	44.9
Total	834,246	24.6	1,074,432	21.7	1,426,508	26.8	1,592,462	27.9

Note: Numbers are weighted to the population.
*1985 and 1990 data are not available for chronic conditions.

Figure 7.4 Percentage of Canadian Population with Hypertension by 5-Year Age Groups, Females, 1978/79–2000/01

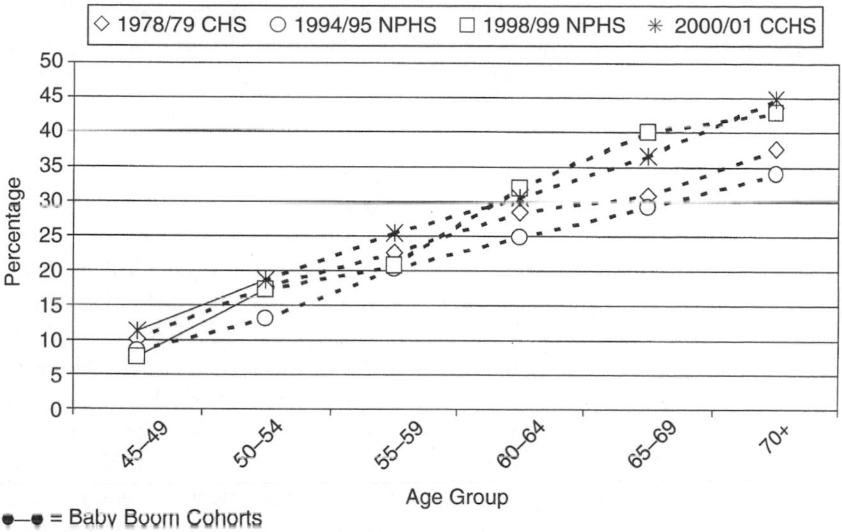

●—● = Baby Boom Cohorts

Note: 1985 and 1990 data are not available for chronic conditions.

linear trend from 11.5% for men aged 45 to 49 to 34.8% for men aged 70 and over. It is also apparent that the largest increase in hypertension between 1978/79 and 2000/01 has occurred for men over the age of 55 at those periods.

Some Concerning Trends in Hypertension for Women

The hypertension rates for women aged 45 and over are actually higher than for men, and exhibit an upward trajectory over the last decade (see bottom row, Table 7.4). In 1978/79, the hypertension rate for all women aged 45 and over is 24.6%. The 1994/95 rate dropped to 21.7%, but rose significantly in 1998/99 to 26.8%, and in 2000/01 to 27.9%. The relative percentage change in these rates shows a decrease of 12% between 1978/79 and 1994/95, but an increase of 29% between 1994/95 and 2000/01. It can be observed as well that the rise in the female hypertension rate is more prevalent among older women aged 60 and over, as seen in Figure 7.4. Furthermore, the upturn in the hypertension rate among women aged 45 and over is sharper than observed for men. For example, in 2000/01 women aged 45 to 49 had a rate of only 11.3%, which builds to an alarming 44.9% among women 70 and over. In addition, while men and women aged 45 to 49 report similar hypertension rates in 2000/01, the age-specific rates for women exhibit a steeper incline than for men after age 60. Moreover, their rate is significantly higher (about a 10 percentage point difference) in older age – 34.8% for men aged 70 and beyond in 2000/01, compared to 44.9% for women of that age. These differences underline the importance of viewing hypertension, as well as heart disease, as illness that influences both sexes and not just men – a common misperception in past years.

Arthritis for Men: Still an Old-Age Problem

The prevalence rates of arthritis are presented for persons aged 40 and over, based on the earlier onset of this condition compared to hypertension. It can be seen in Table 7.5 (bottom row) that no appreciable change has occurred for rates of arthritis for men over the age of 40 for the time period under observation. The arthritis rate is 21.4% in 1978/79, 19.2% in 1994.95, 21.1% in 1998/99, and 20.7 in 2000/01. However, a distinct aging pattern occurs for the prevalence of arthritis (see Figure 7.5). For example, in 2000/01 the arthritis rate inflates from 8.1% for men aged 40 to 44 to 35.6% for those aged 70 and over. Thus, arthritis appears to be an aging-related problem that is not significantly shaped by period or cohort effects.

Higher Prevalence of Arthritis in Women

Similar to the period pattern for men, Table 7.6 indicates that there has been little or no systematic change in the rate of arthritis for women over time. The bottom row of this table reveals that the arthritis rate for women 40 and over is 34.1% in 1978/79, 28.7% in 1994/95, 34.5% in 1998/99, and 32.5% in 2000/01. Yet, once again, the most prominent trend is the upturn in arthritis that occurs as people age (see Figure 7.6). For example, in 2000/01 the arthritis rate slopes upward, from 12.8% for women aged 40 to 44 to 53.2% for those aged 70 and beyond.

Another important pattern is the gender difference for arthritis – the prevalence of arthritis is 1.5 to 2 times higher for women than for men. For instance, in 2000/01 the arthritis rate is 8.1% for men aged 40 to 44, but 12.8% for women of that age. For persons aged 70 and over in that year, the rate is reported to be 35.6% for men (about 1/3 of the population) and 53.2% for women (more than half). Thus, arthritis rates tend to rise fairly rapidly as people move through late adulthood and into their senior years, they apparently have not changed much over the last two decades, and women report this chronic condition at considerably higher rates than men.

Table 7.5
Percentage of Canadian Population with Arthritis, Males 40+, 1978/79–2000/01*

	Survey							
	1978/79 CHS		1994/95 NPHS		1998/99 NPHS		2000/01 CCHS	
Age Group	N	%	N	%	N	%	N	%
40–44	32,924	5.3	69,006	6.0	88,688	6.4	110,237	8.1
45–49	69,054	11.1	83,007	8.1	114,404	11.4	131,409	11.3
50–54	111,126	18.8	105,526	13.3	125,731	13.3	155,042	15.2
55–59	118,948	22.4	114,777	19.2	141,932	19.6	170,473	21.3
60–64	110,990	25.9	119,794	21.7	184,272	29.3	149,320	24.8
65–69	123,032	34.5	160,288	30.6	147,987	29.9	155,372	28.3
70+	167,099	31.5	307,866	35.3	389,165	38.2	370,983	35.6
Total	733,173	21.4	960,264	19.2	1,192,179	21.2	1,242,836	20.7

Note: Numbers are weighted to the population.
*1985 and 1990 data are not available for chronic conditions.

Table 7.6
Percentage of Canadian Population with Arthritis, Females 40+, 1978/79–2000/01*

| | Survey | | | | | | | |
| Age Group | 1978/79 CHS | | 1994/95 NPHS | | 1998/99 NPHS | | 2000/01 CCHS | |
	N	%	N	%	N	%	N	%
40–44	89,577	14.5	105,833	9.5	167,181	13.0	172,838	12.8
45–49	122,970	19.9	130,922	13.9	198,431	17.9	204,828	17.0
50–54	162,193	26.5	168,048	22.6	248,053	26.9	263,945	25.6
55–59	206,245	35.7	210,083	30.7	241,008	37.3	270,997	34.6
60–64	203,196	42.9	222,021	35.7	310,100	44.9	252,307	39.4
65–69	188,325	46.4	236,982	40.8	288,038	47.6	270,465	45.0
70+	383,147	52.8	607,442	47.9	737,734	54.1	769,082	53.2
Total	1,355,653	34.1	1,681,331	28.7	2,190,545	34.5	2,204,462	32.5

Note: Numbers are weighted to the population.
*1985 and 1990 data are not available for chronic conditions.

Figure 7.5 Percentage of Canadian Population with Arthritis by 5-Year Age Groups, Males, 1978/79–2000/01

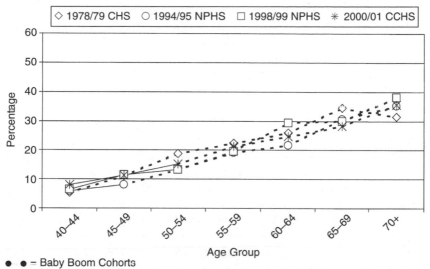

● ● = Baby Boom Cohorts

Note: 1985 and 1990 data are not available for chronic conditions.

Figure 7.6 Percentage of Canadian Population with Arthritis by 5-Year Age Groups, Females, 1978/79–2000/01

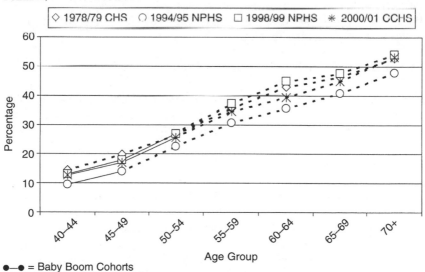

●—● = Baby Boom Cohorts

Note: 1985 and 1990 data are not available for chronic conditions.

A National Concern: Trends in Diabetes for Men

Diabetes is another major chronic illness affecting the Canadian population and one that has been directly linked, in earlier chapters, to rising rates of obesity. Table 7.7 displays rates of diabetes for males aged 45 and over. This age range is again selected because of relatively low prevalence rates of diabetes among persons under age 45, at least until very recently. The bottom row of Table 7.7 demonstrates that the diabetes rate for men aged 45 and over doubled in 22 years. The diabetes rate for all men 45 and over is reported to be 4.1% in 1978/79, 7.1% in 1994/95, 8.2% in 1998/99, and 9.8% in 2000/01. Furthermore, Figure 7.7 shows that in relative terms (percentage change), this increase has occurred fairly uniformly across all ages, except for men 70 and beyond, who have experienced the highest increase. For example, there is a 125% percentage increase in diabetes between 1978/79 and 2000/01 for men aged 45 to 49, and a 92% rise for those aged 60 to 64, but a remarkable 190% increase among men aged 70 and over for the same period. There is also a strong incline in diabetes prevalence across the age groups comprising the lifespan. As can be seen in 2000/01, the diabetes rate is 3.6% among men aged 45 to 49 and 5.7% among men aged 50 to 54; however, it jumps to an alarming 9.1% among men aged 55 to 59, 11.5% among men aged 60 to 64, 14% among men aged 65 to 69, and reaches a high of 15.1% among men 70 and over (also see Figure 7.7). Thus, the prevalence of diabetes shows a strong age-specific pattern, increasing rapidly across age groups. Diabetes appears to be on the rise for males of all ages (but especially middle-aged men aged 45 to 49), and seems to be tracking obesity rates.

Slower Upward Trends in Diabetes for Women

A more gradual but significant progression in the prevalence of diabetes can be observed in Table 7.8 (bottom row) for women aged 45 and over. The diabetes rate for all women of this age is 4.6% in 1978/79, 6.1% in 1994/95, 6.4% in 1998/99, and 7.4% in 2000/01 (also see Figure 7.8). Although the diabetes rate has risen between 1978/79 and 2000/01 for all age groups, there is some fluctuation. It is noteworthy that for women, the highest percentage increase in diabetes occurred for women aged 45 to 49. Specifically, there is a striking 147% percentage jump in diabetes between 1978/79 and 2000/01 for women aged 45 to 49, but only a 52% rise for those aged 60 to 64, and a 54% increase for women aged 70 and over for the same period. Note that women aged 45 to 49 comprise part of the baby boom generation in 2000/01 (also see Chapter 8). Additionally, it is obvious from examining Figure 7.8 that the diabetes rate for

Table 7.7

Percentage of Canadian Population with Diabetes, Males 45+, 1978/79–2000/01*

	Survey								
	1978/79 CHS		1994/95 NPHS		1998/99 NPHS		2000/01 CCHS	
Age Group	N	%	N	%	N	%	N	%
45–49	9,690	1.6	14,776	1.4	35,009	3.5	42,034	3.6
50–54	15,385	2.6	38,326	4.8	35,457	3.7	58,049	5.7
55–59	14,931	2.8	54,063	9.0	48,422	6.7	72,518	9.1
60–64	25,729	6.0	25,638	4.7	58,887	9.4	68,857	11.5
65–69	21,662	6.1	56,673	10.8	50,614	10.2	76,656	14.0
70+	27,767	5.2	120,723	13.8	158,368	15.5	157,950	15.1
Total	115,164	4.1	310,199	7.1	386,757	8.2	476,064	9.8

Note: Numbers are weighted to the population.
*1985 and 1990 data are not available for chronic conditions.

Table 7.8
Percentage of Canadian Population with Diabetes, Females 45+, 1978/79–2000/01*

Age Group	Survey							
	1985 HPS*		1990 HPS		1994/95 NPHS		2000/01 CCHS	
	N	%	N	%	N	%	N	%
45–49	9,479	1.5	17,953	1.9	39,465	3.6	44,601	3.7
50–54	21,081	3.4	14,581	2.0	23,993	2.6	44,957	4.4
55–59	19,188	3.3	41,767	6.1	37,838	5.8	49,989	6.4
60–64	26,431	5.6	36,656	5.9	44,062	6.4	54,480	8.5
65–69	24,771	6.1	57,889	10.0	64,939	10.7	57,932	9.6
70+	55,519	7.6	128,058	10.1	126,188	9.3	169,818	11.7
Total	156,469	4.6	296,904	6.1	336,485	6.4	421,777	7.4

Note: Numbers are weighted to the population.
*1985 and 1990 data are not available for chronic conditions.

Figure 7.7 Percentage of Canadian Population with Diabetes by 5-Year Age Groups, Males, 1978/79–2000/01

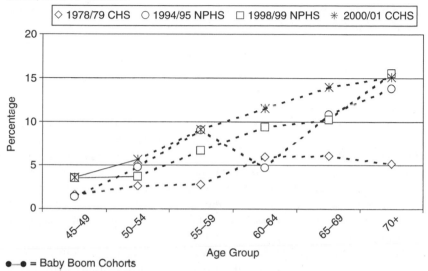

●—● = Baby Boom Cohorts

Note: 1985 and 1990 data are not available for chronic conditions.

Figure 7.8 Percentage of Canadian Population with Diabetes by 5-Year Age Groups, Females, 1978/79–2000/01

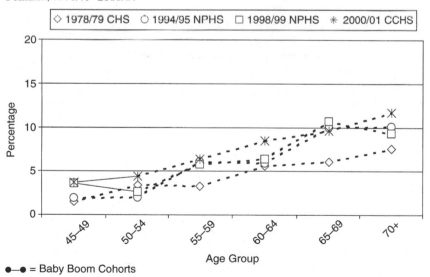

●—● = Baby Boom Cohorts

Note: 1985 and 1990 data are not available for chronic conditions.

women generally builds slower over the age span than for men, and does not reach the same level – about 15% prevalence for men and 12% for women. These patterns mirror those for obesity, raising concerns about the quality and quantity of food intake and the physical activity levels of Canadians, issues to be discussed in detail in Chapter 11.

Trends in Doctor Visits for Men

We turn now to a key measure of health utilization: doctor visits. Since most Canadians see their family physician or general practitioner once or twice in a given year for routine exams, it was decided to present rates of three or more visits to a doctor (of any type) per year. It is assumed that this will provide a crude but useful indicator to identify population trends with regard to doctor visits. We supplement these data with trends in average doctor visits. Table 7.9 and Figure 7.9 show these rates, of three or more visits, for males 15 and over for four surveys between 1978/79 and 2000/01. It is observed that there has been a significant elevation in physician visits between the late 1970s and the 1990s, but that the rate of such visits has remained relatively constant more recently. In 1978/79, 27.9% of males aged 15 or more reported three or more visits to medical doctors in the past year. This rose to 43.5% in 1994/95, dropped slightly to 42.8% in 1998/99, and went up to 44.7% in 2000/01. The increase in doctor visits has been experienced for each age group, and the general pattern across the life cycle has remained similar for the various survey years. Specifically, doctor visits rise gradually over the age span until about age 50, at which time a steeper incline in the rate occurs. In 2000/01, for example, the rate of seeing a medical doctor three or more times a year is 37.9% for males aged 15 to 19, 45.9% for those 50 to 54, 55.5% for those 55 to 59, and 77.3% for persons 70 plus (also see Figure 7.9). It is also noteworthy that the front end of the baby boom generation is in the 50- to 54-year age group in 2000/01, the point at which the number of doctor visits shifts upward.

As can be seen in Figure 7.9, the upturn in doctor visits between 1978/79 and 2000/01 has occurred for all age groups. Calculations of relative percent-age change demonstrates that, for all but one age group, the relative increase in the rate of three or more doctor visits is approximately between 35% and 45%. The one exception is a 97% increase, or a doubling of the rate, for males aged 15 to 19 between 1978/79 and 2000/01, rising from a prevalence of 19.2% in 1978/79 to 37.9% in 2000/01. This indicates that, while a general pattern of more doctor visits per year is occurring, this trend seems to have been magnified for young males prior to moving into an adult status.

To supplement these data, the average number of self-reported doctor visits

Table 7.9

Percentage of Canadian Population Reporting 3+ Doctor Visits in the Past 12 Months by 5-Year Age Groups, Males, 1978/79–2000/01*

	Survey							
	1978/79 CHS		1994/95 NPHS		1998/99 NPHS		2000/01 CCHS	
Age Group	N	%	N	%	N	%	N	%
15–19	227,670	19.2	380,613	36.0	302,505	27.8	412,073	37.9
20–24	264,303	24.2	288,620	34.7	308,238	31.8	356,188	33.3
25–29	219,490	22.4	344,934	31.9	313,031	33.5	303,305	30.0
30–34	164,656	18.3	458,300	36.6	376,030	34.2	370,485	34.0
35–39	167,318	23.7	502,885	38.1	567,009	41.7	475,082	37.3
40–44	154,479	25.2	434,118	37.7	509,616	37.1	524,438	38.7
45–49	170,301	27.5	401,916	39.4	387,485	38.5	510,993	43.9
50–54	184,084	31.5	383,436	48.3	407,364	43.0	466,602	45.9
55–59	178,809	33.8	307,629	51.5	386,439	53.4	442,673	55.5
60–64	205,879	48.6	304,582	55.3	348,394	55.3	370,963	61.6
65–69	154,905	43.8	349,593	67.2	300,145	61.0	352,884	64.4
70+	286,509	54.4	644,225	73.8	782,957	76.8	799,578	77.3
Total	2,378,403	27.9	4,800,951	43.5	4,989,213	42.8	5,385,264	44.7

Note: Numbers are weighted to the population.

*1985 and 1990 data are not available for doctor visits.

Figure 7.9 Percentage of Canadian Population Reporting 3+ Doctor Visits in the Past 12 Months by 5-Year Age Groups, Males, 1978/79–2000/01

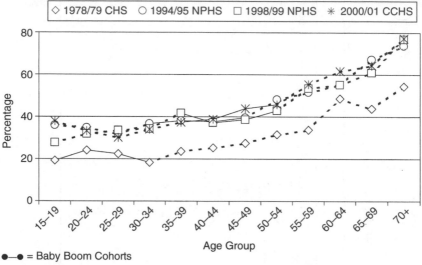

●—● = Baby Boom Cohorts

Note: 1985 and 1990 data are not available for chronic conditions.

has been calculated and is presented in Table 7.9a. Here we observe that the average number of doctor visits for males 15 and over rose from 3.70 in 1978/ 79 to 5.03 in 1994/95, dropped slightly to 4.86 in 1998/99, and declined even further to 3.78 in 2000/01. These trends parallel the ones noted above, showing a peak in doctor visits in the mid-1990s.

Trends in Doctor Visits for Women

As observed in Table 7.10, the rate of seeing a doctor three or more times in the past year also rose over this period for women. In 1978/79, 44.2% of all females aged 15 and over visited a medical doctor three or more times in the previous year. This went up to 61.4% in 1994/95 and 62.5% in 1998/99, then dropped slightly to 62.1% in 2000/01. Similar to men, the increase was reported consistently across age groups, including the baby boomers, and tends to be higher for younger women in 2000/01 compared to those of that age in the late '70s. Specifically, examining the data for 2000/01, we observe that 55.7% of females aged 15 to 19 reported three or more visits a year. This rate hovers around the 55% to 60% level until the 50s, at which point it

Table 7.9a
Mean Number of Doctor Visits in the Past 12 Months, Males, 1978/79–2000/01

Age Group	Survey			
	1978/79 CHS	1994/95 NPHS	1998/99 NPHS	2000/01 CCHS
15–19	2.79	3.94	3.32	2.86
20–24	2.98	3.61	3.12	2.61
25–29	2.89	3.55	3.88	2.66
30–34	2.72	4.30	3.70	2.87
35–39	2.76	4.30	4.06	3.12
40–44	3.59	4.67	4.30	3.29
45–49	3.80	4.96	4.55	3.69
50–54	4.09	5.21	5.07	3.81
55–59	4.44	5.70	5.26	4.60
60–64	5.37	6.07	5.58	5.31
65–69	5.37	6.40	6.15	5.59
70+	5.80	7.54	7.86	6.99
Total	3.70	5.03	4.86	3.78

*1985 and 1990 data are not available for doctor visits.

begins to rise, to a high of 77.8% for women aged 70 and over. As expected, there is an upturn in this rate around the childbearing years for women (see Figure 7.10).

It can also be noted that the relative percentage change in doctor visits repeats the pattern for men. For all ages (except 15–19), there has been a 30% to 40% relative increase between 1978/79 and 2000/01, whereas for females aged 15 to19, there has been a striking 85% jump. Thus, while the rise in physician utilization appears to be relatively consistent across all age groups for men and women, teenagers stand out as the exception.

Furthermore, while men and women report similar rates by the time that they reach their elder years (see Tables 7.9 and 7.10), women start off higher than men and continue this trajectory across the earlier stages of the life span, resulting in an overall or total rate that is *one-third higher* (62.1% compared to only 44.7%). By comparing Figures 7.9 and 7.10, it can be ascertained also that visiting a doctor three or more times a year is common for even young women (about 60%), whereas the percentage is about one-third for teenage males 15 to 19. Furthermore, males do not reach the 60% mark until about age

Table 7.10
Percentage of Canadian Population Reporting 3+ Doctor Visits in the Past 12 Months by 5-Year Age Groups, Females, 1978/79–2000/01*

| | Survey | | | | | | | |
| | 1978/79 CHS | | 1994/95 NPHS | | 1998/99 NPHS | | 2000/01 CCHS | |
Age Group	N	%	N	%	N	%	N	%
15–19	342,179	30.1	543,184	55.0	572,214	54.6	578,215	55.7
20–24	502,021	45.8	532,664	59.8	634,572	66.5	629,205	60.7
25–29	527,708	52.7	718,423	68.1	506,054	58.0	626,310	63.3
30–34	376,030	41.7	787,625	58.0	735,814	60.9	637,823	60.0
35–39	253,742	35.6	719,288	56.6	809,222	57.8	724,694	55.4
40–44	251,454	41.1	633,961	56.8	676,008	52.7	754,743	56.0
45–49	239,522	39.0	518,807	55.1	650,216	58.8	690,731	57.6
50–54	269,595	44.4	457,599	61.7	585,661	63.6	650,845	63.3
55–59	270,954	47.3	422,133	62.2	445,344	69.2	500,147	63.8
60–64	236,924	50.2	409,512	65.5	450,741	65.4	425,808	66.6
65–69	226,832	56.3	424,046	73.0	433,330	71.7	410,422	68.5
70+	413,476	57.2	898,682	71.2	1,052,246	77.3	1,119,215	77.8
Total	3,910,437	44.2	7,065,924	61.4	7,551,422	62.5	7,748,158	62.1

Note: Numbers are weighted to the population.
*1985 and 1990 data are not available for doctor visits.

Figure 7.10 Percentage of Canadian Population Reporting 3+ Doctor Visits in the Past
12 Months by 5-Year Age Groups, Females, 1978/79–2000/01

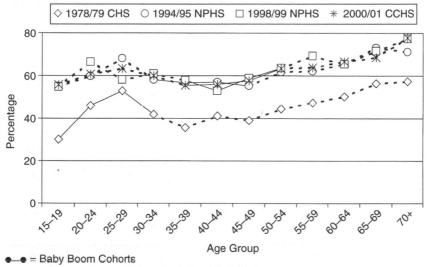

●—● = Baby Boom Cohorts

Note: 1985 and 1990 data are not available for chronic conditions.

60 to 64. These trends are consistent with literature pertaining to gender
differences in doctor visits, as well as to other health utilization measures. Part
of this gender difference is due no doubt, to the higher intensity of doctor visits
during the childbearing years and visits pertaining to contraception use, but it
can be seen in the five-year age data that the period in life at which time this
occurs (20–44) only accounts for some of the total gender difference.

Adding to these analyses, Table 7.10a exhibits the average number of doctor
visits reported by females. These rates are higher than for males, but generally
reflect a similar upward pattern between 1978/79 and the mid-1990s, followed
by a slight downturn. The average number of doctor visits is reported as 4.80
in 1978/79, 6.53 in 1994/95, 6.01 in 1998/99, and 5.40 in 2000/01.

Overall, the pattern of three of more annual doctor visits has risen appreciably since the late 1970s; however, it is also apparent that it may have peaked,
or at least reached a threshold, in the mid-1990s. Thus, although the number of
chronic conditions has steadily increased, doctor visits have reached a high
point in the mid-1990s and may actually be on the decline since that time. It is
likely that shrinkages to the health care budgets of many provinces during the

Table 7.10a
Mean Number of Doctor Visits in the Past 12 Months, Females, 1978/79–2000/01

Age Group	Survey			
	1978/79 CHS	1994/95 NPHS	1998/99 NPHS	2000/01 CCHS
15–19	3.57	5.81	4.88	4.44
20–24	4.58	7.07	6.15	5.15
25–29	5.34	6.91	6.06	5.72
30–34	4.54	6.49	5.79	5.43
35–39	3.82	6.28	5.59	5.03
40–44	4.24	5.71	5.04	4.81
45–49	4.59	6.30	5.16	4.90
50–54	5.10	6.04	6.31	5.47
55–59	4.75	5.96	6.31	5.55
60–64	5.52	6.02	6.12	5.68
65–69	5.68	7.06	6.17	5.75
70+	6.60	7.44	7.33	6.98
Total	4.80	6.53	6.01	5.40

*1985 and 1990 data are not available for doctor visits.

1990s have resulted in a concomitant drop in utilization. Finally, fairly striking gender differences persist. The most prominent that is observed over the two decades appears to be for teenage males and females, where it can be seen that teenage females receive considerably more physician care than males.

8

Comparative Health Dynamics of Baby Boomers

Introduction

This chapter focuses specifically on the baby boomers in an effort to identify major shifts in health behaviours, chronic conditions, and health utilization as these individuals move up the age escalator. The primary purpose of this analysis is to determine how well baby boomers are aging in midlife by comparing their health dynamics against persons of the same age in earlier periods. This also will allow for predictions about future health care demands in Canada. We selected two 10-year age groups approximating younger and older baby boomers. Although this division is arbitrary, it allows for separation of the baby boom generation into two equal age groupings for more detailed comparisons. If linked to the latest survey date (set at 2000), persons aged approximately 35 to 44 constitute younger baby boomers and those aged 45 to 54 constitute older ones. Using the year 2000 as a benchmark, younger baby boomers (aged 35–44 in 2000) were born between 1956 and 1965, whereas older baby boomers (aged 45–54 in 2000) were born between 1946 and 1955. Since the Canadian Community Health Survey was collected in both 2000 and 2001, our definition of the baby boom generation (born between 1946 and 1965) is not a perfect match with the standard five- and 10-year age groups used. However, approximately 95% of the baby boom generation, as defined in this book, will be included when using these age groups.

As a starting point for each section, data are also presented for the combined age groups (35–54), reflecting midlife health patterns for the full baby boom generation. Thus, we can compare trends (period effects) in health dynamics between 1978/79 and 2000/01 to ascertain whether and to what extent baby boomers are exhibiting better health profiles compared to persons of the same age at different points in time. The furthest points cover 22 years on average, or about two decades, which can be considered a generation apart. This analysis will be followed by an examination of whether the patterns are relatively similar for younger versus older baby boomers. Thus, only a partial age-period-cohort analysis is possible because we are studying only two 10-year age cohorts over the period of study. Gender differences are not included in this analysis due to overlap with earlier analyses. As a reminder, Tables 5.7 and 5.8 in Chapter 5 provide the age of the individual baby boomer birth cohorts at each survey date. We again examine percentage change as well as percentage point differences to elucidate key trends. In addition to the use of confidence intervals, as a rule of thumb, percentage change fluctuations in a rate or comparisons of rates of less than 5% may be due to sampling error and will be deemed insignificant. The data are presented only as figures; however, the tabular data upon which they are based are compiled in the Appendix.

What Is the Story for Lifestyle Behaviours?

Baby Boomers Smoke Less in Midlife Than Earlier Cohorts

We can see in Figure 8.1 that the smoking rate for the full baby boom generation (persons aged 35–54 in 2000/01) is significantly lower than for persons of those exact ages in earlier periods. In fact, they exhibit a smoking rate that is 40.4% lower than persons of their age approximately 22 years earlier, in 1978/79. (These data are presented in Table A8.1 in the Appendix.) Indeed, 26.1% of the baby boomers smoked in 2000/01, compared to the following rates for same-aged persons: 43.8% in 1978/79, 32.8% in 1985, 31% in 1990, and 28.7% in 1994/95. Also apparent in these data is the fact that, even if we adjust for the slightly wider period between the 1978/79 and 1985 surveys, the lion's share of the decline in smoking occurred during that time. The late 1970s and early 1980s was without a doubt a period when lifestyles improved the most, including reductions in smoking rates.

Furthermore, there is a slightly larger drop in smoking among older baby boomers than younger ones compared to persons their exact age two decades earlier. Figure 8.1 juxtaposes persons aged 35 to 44 in 1978/79 with our group of younger boomers (aged 35–44 in 2000/01), portraying a decline in smoking from 43.8% to 27.2% (a relative decrease of 37.9%). Turning to comparisons between older and younger boomers, the relative decrease in the smoking rate across the generations is about equal.

Figure 8.1 Percentage of Regular Smokers Aged 35–54 in 5 Canadian Health Surveys, 1978/79–2000/01

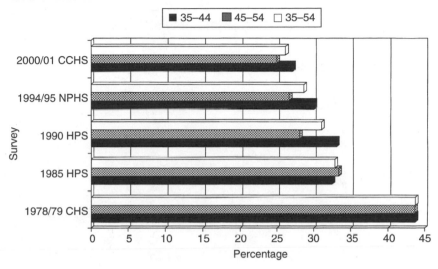

Baby Boomers Are Less Sedentary Than Earlier Cohorts

Interestingly, Figure 8.2 presents a very similar trend to the one observed for smoking for the percentage of persons who are sedentary or infrequent exercisers – what we again call unhealthy exercise. Overall, the percentage of baby boomers that were engaging in unhealthy exercise was 40.9% lower in relative terms than for midlife Canadians a little more than two decades earlier. In 2000/01, only 39.3% of persons aged 35 to 54 were unhealthy in their exercise level, but a striking 66.5% were in this category in 1978/79 (see Appendix, Table A8.2). The rates for the interim years are 50.4% in 1985, 55.3% in 1990, and 47.2% in 1994/95. These trends demonstrate that the deflation in unhealthy exercise has been the greatest between 1978/79 and 1985 (even adjusting for the slightly longer period), just as it had for smoking. Moreover, as reported in the exercise levels of the total population in Chapter 6, there has been a reversal in this trend that took place around 1990 (see Figure 8.2). Thus, we appear to have lost about a decade of improvement in exercise, and this has occurred for the baby boomers as well as for most other age groups shown in Chapter 6. On a more positive note, it is also apparent that new watermarks are being made in 2000/01, a point in time at which unhealthy exercise levels are

Figure 8.2 Percentage of Persons Who Are Sedentary or Infrequent Exercisers*
Aged 35–54 in 5 Canadian Health Surveys, 1978/79–2000/01

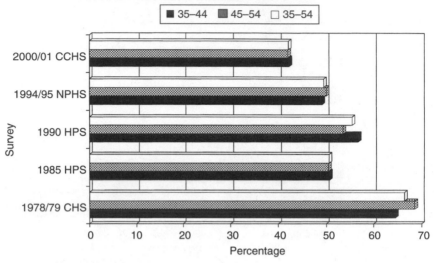

*15 min. of physical activity <3X per week.

at an all-time low, and, conversely, healthy exercise levels are at an all-time
high. Yet, there can be little celebration among baby boomers when approximately 40% do not meet minimum exercise levels. In this respect, baby
boomers mirror virtually all other age groups in Canadian society.

Comparisons of declines in unhealthy exercise over the two-decade period
for the younger and older baby boomers again show no significant differences.
Thus, the improvement in physical activity involves younger and older baby
boomers equally.

Baby Boomers Are More Obese Than Earlier Cohorts

In sharp contrast, Figure 8.3 indicates that baby boomers are not exhibiting a
healthy lifestyle in terms of body mass index. Indeed, obesity rates have
doubled over the 15-year period between the surveys for which BMI measures
are available – 1985 and 2000/01. Note that the 1978/79 data are not reliable
because BMI was only collected for a subset of the population and therefore
have been omitted. For the total complement of baby boomers aged 35 to 54 in
the most recent survey period, the obesity rate is 16.2%, but it is only 8.2% for

Figure 8.3 Percentage of Persons Aged 35–54 Who Are Obese (BMI 30+) in 4 Canadian Health Surveys, 1985–2000/01

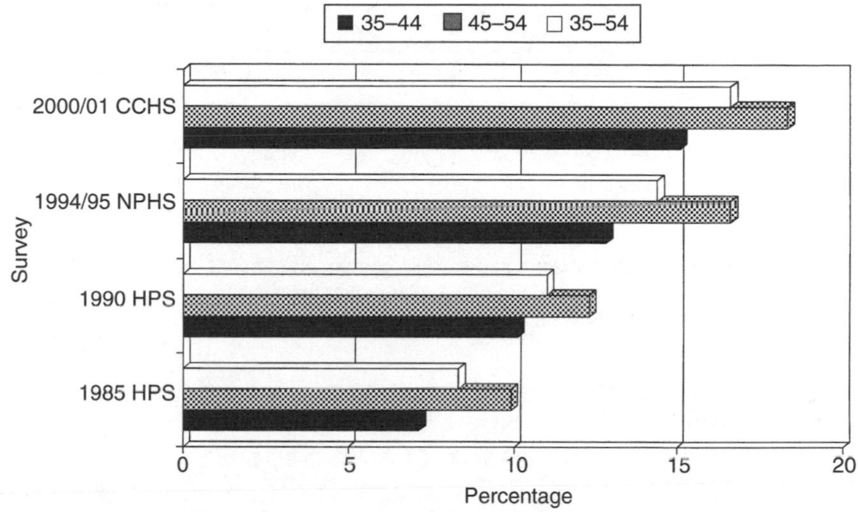

Noto: Since DMI was collected for only a 20% sub-sample of the 1978/79 CHS, the population estimates are unreliable and have been omitted.

similarly aged persons in 1985 (rates shown in Table A8.3, Appendix). The rates are 10.9% in 1990 and 14.1% in 1994/95 for midlife Canadians of the same age. Furthermore, the bulge in obesity rates is slightly higher for younger baby boomers (110% increase) than for older baby boomers (86% increase), a 24% difference in the relative rise in obesity between younger and older boomers.

A similar but less pronounced pattern is apparent for mean levels of BMI, shown only in tabular form in Table 8.1. The mean BMI for baby boomers aged 35 to 54 in 2000/01 is shown to be 25.88 compared to 24.49 for persons that age in 1985. This has pushed midlife baby boomers to an average BMI that is fast approaching the threshold for being overweight, that is, a body mass index of 27 or higher.

Baby Boomers Drink Less Than Earlier Cohorts

Figure 8.4 shows that only 6.3% of baby boomers in midlife (aged 35–54) in 2000/01 reported heavy drinking, compared to 13.8% of persons of that age in 1978/79 (rates shown in Table A8.4, Appendix). This represents a 54.3%

Table 8.1
Mean BMI of the Canadian Population Aged 35–54, 1985–2000/01*

	Age Group		
Survey	35–44	45–54	35–54
1985 HPS	24.15	24.97	24.49
1990 HPS	24.78	25.30	24.99
1994/95 NPHS	25.18	26.17	25.59
2000/01 CCHS	25.54	26.30	25.88

*Since BMI was collected only for a sub-sample composed of about
20% of the 1978/79 CHS sample, the population estimates are
unreliable and have been omitted.

Figure 8.4 Percentage of Heavy Drinkers* Aged 35–54 in 5 Canadian Health Surveys,
1978/79–2000/01

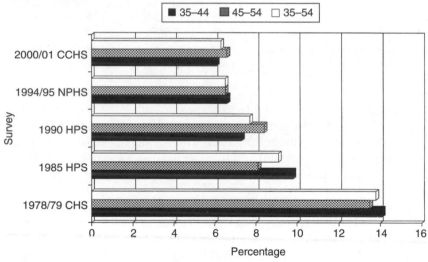

*Males = 14+ drinks/week; females = 12+ drinks/week.

decrease in rates of heavy drinking comparing baby boomers in 2000/01 to
persons of that same age in 1978/79. Furthermore, we note rates of heavy
drinking at 9% in 1985, 7.7% in 1990, and 6.5% in 1994/95. Again, the
greatest decline in heavy drinking has also occurred between 1978/79 and
1985. Interestingly, the younger baby boomers have experienced a slightly
larger drop in the rate of heavy drinking over this period (57.4% decrease) than

older baby boomers (51% decrease), but this 6.4% relative difference is negligible.

Multiple Healthy Lifestyle Behaviours of Baby Boomers

Overall, the report card for baby boomers, compared to midlife Canadians of the same age in earlier periods, is both good and bad. Baby boomers have reduced their smoking rate considerably, they have lowered their rate of unhealthy exercise behaviour, and they have lowered their prevalence of heavy drinking. However, the rise in obesity is an obvious failing grade. Moreover, there remains considerable room for further progress even in areas in which there have been declines in unhealthy lifestyle behaviour – especially rates of exercise, given that about four out of ten baby boomers today engage in levels that are below minimum recommended standards, and of smoking, given that one in four smoke.

Some of these patterns coincide with the 1996 Heart and Stroke Foundation of British Columbia and Yukon study presented earlier. It was shown that baby boomers in the early 1990s were doing better in terms of smoking than adults of the same age in the 1970s, but that fewer of the boomers had a healthy blood pressure and a healthy serum cholesterol level. This study departs from ours in that it shows a slight reduction in exercise rates, and, oddly, improved weight. For example, it reports that the percentage of adults in the 1990s who exercise regularly was 35% compared to 38% of adults the same age in the 1970s. The difference in exercise patterns between the two studies could be due to the fact that the Heart and Stroke study uses only two time periods, one of which was in the early 1990s, when exercise levels temporarily fell. The findings concerning weight are unexplainable, given that they are inconsistent with the results of all studies reviewed, including the present one. The Heart and Stroke study also reported that comparative percentages for a healthy blood pressure were 75% for baby boomers in the 1990s and 84% for persons the same age in the 1970s, and that a healthy serum cholesterol level was reported to be 55% and 86%, respectively.

The more detailed analysis comprising the original research in this book also establishes some nuances between older and younger baby boomers. Older baby boomers have exhibited a rise in obesity that has not been as dramatic in relative terms compared to younger baby boomers. However, younger baby boomers have lowered their rate of heavy drinking slightly more than older baby boomers when we compare them to persons of their age two decades earlier. These differences suggest that the baby boom generation should not be considered a homogeneous group, since it obviously is experiencing some unique patterns of unhealthy lifestyles. The relevance of these trends is also embedded in the fact that the baby boomers comprise a third of the total population of Canada, and the front cohorts are fast approaching their elder years. The improvements in smoking, exercise, and heavy drinking should have a positive impact on how this group ages, but the dramatic rise in obesity may wipe out a good portion of the former, especially the effect of obesity on diabetes and cardiovascular disease.

What Is the Picture for Chronic Illnesses?

More Chronic Illnesses among Baby Boomers Than among Earlier Cohorts

Since data on chronic illnesses are not available in the 1985 and 1990 Health Promotion Surveys, we include here the 1998/99 National Population Health data, similar to Chapter 7. Like the earlier chapter, the self-report measure of chronic illness entails the presence of any chronic illness. As observed graphically in Figure 8.5, there has been a 19% relative increase in the percentage of midlife baby boomers aged 35 to 54 reporting a chronic condition in 2000/01 compared to persons that age in 1978/79 (also see Table A8.5, Appendix). However, this has not been a linear trend, since we observe a slight, temporary drop in the chronic illness rate in 1994/95, suggesting some degree of fluctuation. In 1978/79, 53% of persons aged 35 to 54 reported having at least one chronic condition; this dropped to 51.8% in 1994/95, rose to 58.3% in 1998/99, and increased further to 63.1% in 2000/01. Thus, it would appear that the rate of having a chronic illness is rising more rapidly in the 1990s and early 2000s than between the late '70s and the mid-'90s.

We can also observe that the increase is larger and more definitive for younger baby boomers than for older baby boomers compared to midlife individuals their age in earlier periods. Younger boomers aged 35 to 44 in 2000/01 reported a chronic illness rate of 60.1%, which rose from a low of 46.6% in 1978/79 for persons of that age – a 29% rise – whereas the older baby boomers reported a rate of 66.8% in 2000/01 compared to 60% in 1978/79 – an increase of only 11.3%. Thus, compared to persons their age, the younger baby boomers are doing more poorly in terms of the change in self-reported prevalence of chronic illnesses over these two decades than are older boomers. Whether this reflects differences in actual disease, better diagnostics and detection, or a more knowledgeable population is debatable. However, there appears to be a general pattern of relative disadvantage among young boomers compared to older ones in terms of changes in chronic illness when juxtaposed

Figure 8.5 Percentage of Persons Aged 35–54 with a Chronic Condition in 4 Canadian Health Surveys, 1978/79–2000/01

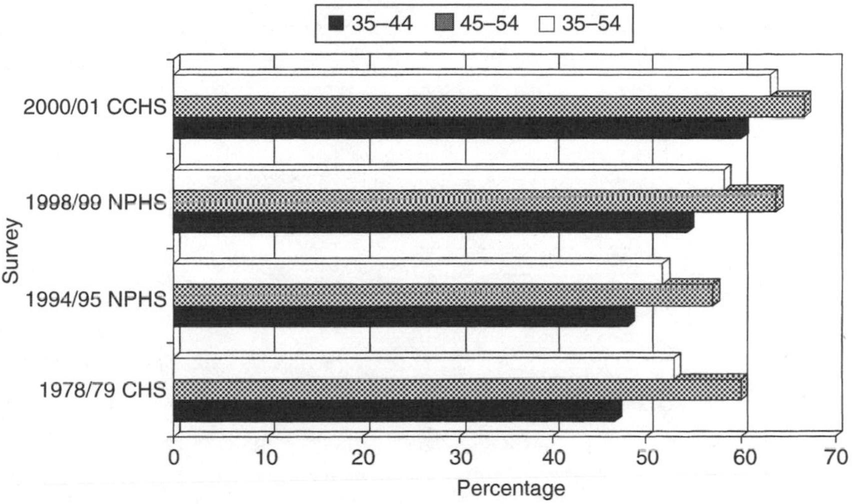

Note: 1985 and 1990 data are not available for chronic conditions.

with persons their age in the late 1970s, many of whom are their parents. We turn now to specific illnesses.

Hypertension Higher among Baby Boomers

Baby boomers in 2000/01 are experiencing rates of hypertension that are slightly higher than persons of their age two decades ago, but the rates have fluctuated again over that period (see Figure 8.6). The hypertension rate among individuals aged 35 to 54 is reported to be 8.1% in 1978/79, declining to 6.6% in 1994/95, then up to 7.5% in 1998/99, and 9.7% in 2000/01 (from data shown in Table A8.6, Appendix). This amounts to a 19.7% rise in hypertension between 1978/79 and 2000/01, suggesting that hypertension has become slightly more prevalent for the boomers, compared to persons their age two decades earlier, and that it continues to be a health problem for about 10% of midlife Canadians aged 35 to 54. Again, a reversal in the trend is seen between 1978/79 and 1994/95. Unfortunately, the absence of illness data in the 1985 and 1990 Health Promotion Surveys do not allow us to pinpoint the actual period in which this reversal takes place. However, based on earlier

Figure 8.6 Percentage of Persons Aged 35–54 with Hypertension in 4 Canadian Health Surveys, 1978/79–2000/01

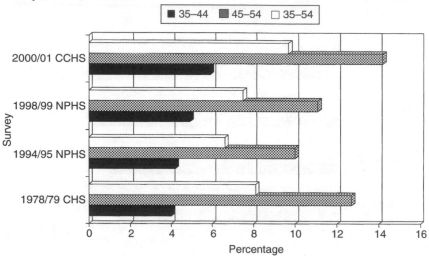

Note: 1985 and 1990 data are not available for chronic conditions.

results, it would seem likely that all Canadians have experienced a number of reversals in health and lifestyle indicators in the late 1980s and/or early 1990s.

Turning to differences within the baby boomer ages, younger baby boomers (persons aged 35–44) exhibit a hypertension rate that has actually increased more than for older baby boomers in relative terms, although absolute rates are obviously lower for younger persons. Between 1978/79 and 2000/01, younger baby boomers, compared to their counterparts, experienced a 47.5% increase in their hypertension rate, whereas the relative change for older boomers is only 11.8%. Whether the incline in hypertension prevalence will translate into higher hypertension rates at older ages is not clear. However, given that high blood pressure is a major risk factor for heart disease, these patterns raise some concern.

Arthritis Also Remains High among Baby Boomers

The situation for arthritis is more promising than for all chronic illness and for hypertension. As seen in Figure 8.7, reported diagnoses of arthritis among persons aged 35 to 54 actually declined between 1978/79 (13.6%) and 2000/01 (12.6%), representing a modest 7.3% drop over the two decades (Table

Figure 8.7 Percentage of Persons Aged 35–54 with Arthritis in 4 Canadian Health
Surveys, 1978/79–2000/01

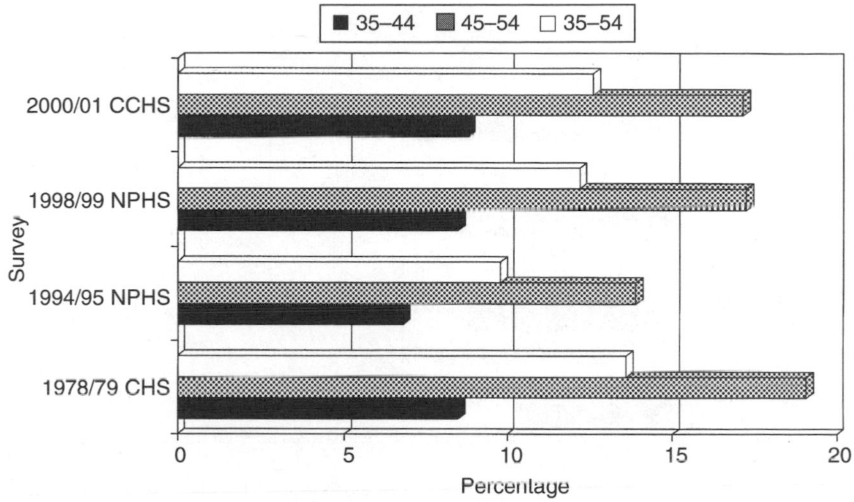

Note: 1985 and 1990 data are not available for chronic conditions.

A8.7, Appendix). In parallel with earlier trends, these rates of arthritis decline
significantly between 1978/79 and 1994/95, followed by an upturn to a point
in 2000/01 that is a bit lower than the starting point in 1978/79. Specifically,
the rates were 13.6% in 1978/79, 9.8% in 1994/95, 12.2% in 1998/99, and
12.6% in 2000/01. This reversal in the trend is apparent for the younger and
older boomers. Also, the entire decline in relative rates of arthritis between
baby boomers in 2000/01 and their counterparts in 1978/79 has occurred for
the older group. This underscores the importance of examining potential
cohort differences within the baby boom generation, and corresponds with the
trend that older baby boomers are fairing better than younger ones compared
to earlier generations.

Rising Rates of Diabetes among Baby Boomers

Probably the most striking pattern in chronic illness in midlife pertains to a
pervasive incline in the rate of diabetes as observed in Figure 8.8. Baby
boomers in 2000/01 have a 76.5% higher rate of diabetes than their counterparts in 1978/79 (drawn from Table A8.8, Appendix). In 1978/79 the rate
was 1.7%, rising to 1.9% in 1994/95, 2.3% in 1998/99, and to a high of 3% in

Figure 8.8 Percentage of Persons Aged 35–54 with Diabetes in 4 Canadian Health Surveys, 1978/79–2000/01

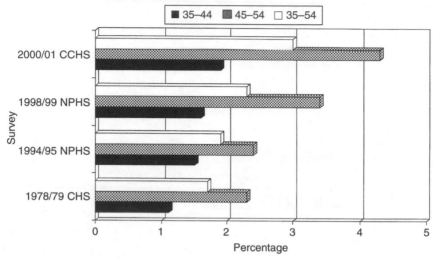

Note: 1985 and 1990 data are not available for chronic conditions.

2000/01. Also, the alarming acceleration in diabetes prevalence appears to have been experienced slightly more among the older baby boomers than for the younger ones; however, diabetes rates for persons in the younger group tend to be very low in general.

Increasing Health Utilization

More Doctor Visits among Baby Boomers

Baby boomers also report more doctor visits (of any type) than persons their age two decades ago, as evidenced in Figure 8.9. In 1978/79, 33.3% of persons aged 35 to 54 reported three or more doctor visits in the past year compared to 48.5% in 1994/95, 48.9% in 1998/99, and 49.5% in 2000/01 (Table A8.9, Appendix). This represents a 48.6% relative increase for the full 22-year period. Today, about half of the baby boomers see a doctor three or more times a year. In addition, these data indicate that the largest rise in doctor visits appears to have taken place during the 1980s and early 1990s, and that over the last six years we seem to be reaching a threshold, or at least the rate of increase appears to be slowing.

Figure 8.9 Percentage of Persons Aged 35–54 with 3+ Doctor Visits in the Past 12 Months in 4 Canadian Health Surveys, 1978/79–2000/01

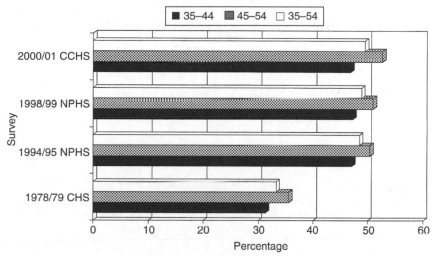

Note: 1905 and 1990 data are not available for doctor visits.

Furthermore, younger and older baby boomers share a similar pattern in doctor visits compared to persons their age in 1978/79. Overall, baby boomers see their doctors three or more times a year at about a 48.6% higher rate than persons their age in the late '70s. This points further to a health care system that has grown in size and treatment intensity over this same period (Barer et al., 1985; Evans et al., 2001).

9

Socio-economic Status, Region, and Foreign-Born Status Variations in Baby Boomer Lifestyles

This chapter examines the lifestyle behaviours of the baby boomers, but with a concentration on socio-economic status, regional, and foreign-born status variations. We begin with socio-economic variables (education and income). This is followed with analyses based on five regions, including the Maritimes, or Atlantic provinces (Newfoundland, Prince Edward Island, Nova Scotia, New Brunswick), Quebec, Ontario, the Prairie provinces (Manitoba, Saskatchewan and Alberta), and British Columbia. Finally, a foreign-born status dichotomy is used to address potential immigration effects on baby boomer health dynamics. It should be noted that all tables mentioned in this chapter can be found in the Appendix. Only the associated figures will be presented in this chapter.

The Socio-economic Status Factor

Socio-economic status (SES) has been established as one of the major determinants of health. People with higher education, income, and occupation, the most commonly used measures of SES, experience longer and healthier lives than those with lower levels (Antonovsky, 1967; Marmot, Kogevinas, and Elston, 1987; Raphael, 2004; Robert and House, 1996; Syme and Berkman, 1979). Part of this effect is manifested through healthier lifestyles among individuals with socio-economic status advantages. Persons with higher education have more prestigious and higher-paid employment, and in turn tend to have more health knowledge, more effectively access health care, and are more likely to have stronger and more stable family and social support systems to develop and sustain healthier lifestyles (Cockerham, Lueschen, Kunz and Spaeth, 1986; Millar, 1996). In addition, individuals with higher levels of education not only have more health knowledge pertaining to the positive influence of healthy lifestyles, but also are more likely to have developed the self-efficacy (confidence) and problem-solving skills that assist in realizing those health goals (Clark, 1996; Mirowsky and Ross, 1998). Coupled with this is the propensity for social capital to be associated with education level, meaning that these individuals tend to enjoy greater benefits associated with connectedness to social networks and communities that may also influence human potential, lifestyle, and health (Berkman and Kawachi, 2000; Coleman, 1988; Lomas, 1998).

Individuals with more disposable income experience more material advantages, such as ability to purchase medicines, more food choices, memberships to various clubs, and better housing, and they tend to live in communities with more lifestyle options (Cockerham et al., 1986; Dunn and Hayes, 2000; Frankel, Speechley, and Wade, 1996; Health Canada, 1994; Robert and House, 1996). Poorer individuals and families more likely experience life stressors associated with financial burden, which is reflected in higher mortality, lower disability-free life expectancy, and less healthy lifestyles (Wilkins and Adams, 1987). Moreover, financial resources have the potential to mitigate life course problems and challenges, such as coping with disabilities. It is also noteworthy that the literature has found that lifestyle behaviours are shaped differently by education and income level (Cockerham et al., 1986; Lock and Wister, 1992.) For example, it has been demonstrated that education is a stronger determinant of healthy exercise than income, whereas the latter tends to influence patterns of smoking (Wister, 1996).

There is also some evidence that socio-economic status is more influential during the middle years of life and that this pattern has been strengthening over time, at least in the United States (Pappas, Queen, Hadden, and Fisher, 1993). This underscores the importance of examining baby boomer health dynamics comparatively by age and by time. However, much remains to be known about the mechanisms that link SES to health, including healthy lifestyle behaviours, both across the life course and across historical time periods.

Population-level improvements in education among successive cohorts therefore would raise the overall health of our population. Indeed, education levels of Canadians have risen consistently over time. For example, the percentage of Canadians with post-secondary education increased more than 54% in two decades, from 30.6% in 1976 to 47.2% in 1996 (Statistics Canada, 1998b). Today, almost half of the adult Canadian population has at least some post-secondary education. These educational trends need to be considered when we examine the consequence of this socio-economic factor on patterns of lifestyle behaviours among persons in midlife. Indeed, many baby boomers have pursued their education over the last three decades and therefore enjoyed the education boom in Canada. The focus on midlife persons aged 35 to 54 is in keeping with the baby boomer theme, since persons this age comprise the baby boomers in 2000/01. These individuals will be compared to persons of the same age for earlier survey dates, which repeats the approach used in Chapter 8.

Like education, the income distribution in a country, as well as changes to that distribution over time, may be an influential determinant of population health. The distribution of total income (in standard dollars) for individuals in Canada has improved during the 1980s and 1990s, however not to the same degree as post-secondary education. The median income of Canadians in 2001 dollars rose 24.6% between 1980 and 2001 (Statistics Canada, 2003). More-over, most of this rise took place during the 1980s (18% between 1980–89, and only 6% between 1990 and 2001). While some groups have made modest progress due to income redistribution policies (e.g., seniors), many groups are still extremely disadvantaged. These include Aboriginals, other visible minorities, single mothers, and unattached older women. Indeed, using medium income converted to real dollars may mask some of the income disparity between the rich and the poor.

Taken together, there has been about a 50% rise in the post-secondary educational level of Canadians over our 22-year period of study (between about 1978 and 2001), but the changes in median income have been about half as large (approximately 24%). It is informative therefore not only to investigate trends in lifestyle factors across these categories of income and education to estimate their influence, but it is also important to estimate the potential ramifications of these associations against population changes in socio-economic status. For example, alterations in the strength of the association between education and smoking over survey periods also needs to be considered against changing post-secondary patterns in society that have taken place. We begin with education differences followed by income for persons aged 35 to 54, which comprises the majority of the baby boomers in 2000/01.

Knowledge Is Health: Educational Differences in Baby Boomer Lifestyles

The following analyses show rates of unhealthy lifestyle behaviours for midlife persons aged 35 to 54 with high school or less, and for those with some or completed post-secondary education. Only these two education categories were used in order to minimize the sampling variability and sampling error associated with the estimates. For the same reason, younger and older baby boomers are not analysed separately. Data are included for five surveys between 1978/79 and 2000/01, except for obesity, where we begin with 1985 data due to availability. Relative percentage differences between education groups (calculated using this formula: high education – low education / low education) are shown in the tables, along with absolute group percentage differences (calculated as simply high education group minus the lower education group), and are discussed where appropriate. Additionally, relative percentage change between the earliest and latest survey years for the education dichotomy are calculated in order to ascertain the extent to which prevalence rates have changed, at different paces, for the two education categories over the two decades. This provides another method to compare systematically the two education groups with respect to their rate changes, within groups, between 1978/79 and 2000/01. It is recognized that this is a simple time-series comparison and that variations may have occurred over this period. Relative percentage differences between education groups that are 5% or larger will be deemed substantively important. Finally, integrating the above findings with the noted population gains in post-secondary education between the late 1970s and 2001 allows for conclusions about investments into education for health behaviours.

Smoking Declines across Education Groups

As graphically shown in Figure 9.1, persons aged 35 to 54 with post-secondary education have lower rates of smoking than those with high school or less for each of the survey years: 1978/79, 1985, 1990, 1994/95, and 2000/01. The group differences in smoking prevalence ranges between 2.1% and 16% lower for the post-secondary or high education group indicated in Table A9.1 (Appendix). In 2000/01, for instance, baby boomers (persons aged 35–54) with post-secondary education reveal a 20.9% smoking rate compared to 34.6% among baby boomers with high school or less – a 13.7 percentage point difference. This amounts to a smoking rate that is more than *one-third lower* for persons with post-secondary education compared to persons with lower education levels. Moreover, the relative difference between the education groups, or the 'education effect,' actually has remained relatively consistent over the time periods, except for 1985.

Furthermore, comparing the column percentages between 1978/79 and 2000/01 in Table A9.1 (Appendix) indicates that the high education group has experienced a slightly greater relative decrease in smoking over this period, although the start and end points are obviously different for each group. Those with post-secondary education experienced a 34.5% relative drop in smoking, and those with high school or less had a 27.8% decline. This suggests that not only is smoking less frequent among more educated midlife Canadians, but

Figure 9.1 Percentage of Canadian Population Aged 35–54 Who Are Regular Smokers by Education Level, 1978/79–2000/01

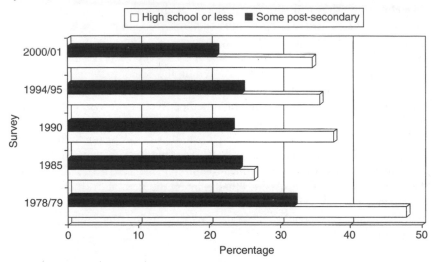

that the decline in smoking rates since the 1970s has been slightly steeper for the more educated.

In addition, as presented earlier, the proportion of the population aged 35 to 54 with some or completed post-secondary education has jumped more than 50% between 1978/79 and 2000/01, from approximately one-third to one-half of the Canadian population. Hence, the upward shift in education level of midlife Canadians over these decades probably has contributed to the decline in smoking at a population level, given the persistent education factor over this period.

Overall, education constitutes a potent determinant of health. It clearly deters smoking and has continued to do so over the last two decades. Moreover, since the education effect is portrayed in these data in a conservative manner because we are simply dividing the population into only two groups, its influence may be muted. For example, comparisons of midlife persons not completing high school with those completing post-secondary programs would result in significantly larger differences in smoking rates. However, the education dichotomy examined here demonstrates unequivocally that education is a strong factor influencing smoking rates, both at individual and population levels. It also provides us with a clear policy implication – raising post-secondary enrolment.

Figure 9.2   Percentage of Canadian Population Aged 35–54 Who Are Sedentary or Infrequent Exercisers* by Education Level, 1978/79–2000/01

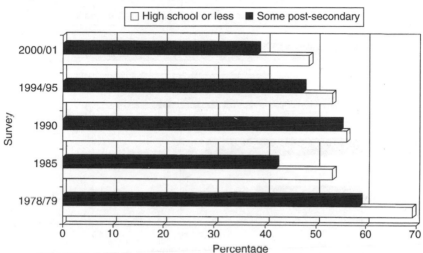

*15 min. of physical activity <3X per week.

Unhealthy Exercise Trends and Education Level

The percentage of the population aged 35 to 54 who do not maintain the minimum guidelines for exercise are also disaggregated for high school or less and for post-secondary education categories in Figure 9.2. The prevalence rate of this unhealthy exercise is consistently lower for persons with post-secondary education than for those with less than this education level, but the difference is smaller than for smoking. For example, in 2000/01, 48.6% of baby boom-aged persons with high school education or less exhibited a poor exercise regiment, whereas only 38.2% of baby boomers with post-secondary education reported unhealthy activity levels (a 21.4% lower rate). This education differential is modest and relatively stable across the survey dates, except for 1990, where we observe a negligible difference (see Table A9.2, Appendix). Additionally, the decline was similar for both education groups.

Since the proportion of individuals completing high school has risen for each successive cohort over the time period under study, it can be assumed that there has been a positive and moderate population health effect of education on exercise. In other words, the expanded access into post-secondary education over the last few decades for baby boomers, coupled with a persistent education effect, has contributed to a more active and healthier population.

Figure 9.3 Percentage of Canadian Population Aged 35–54 Who Are Obese (BMI 30+) by Education Level, 1985–2000/01*

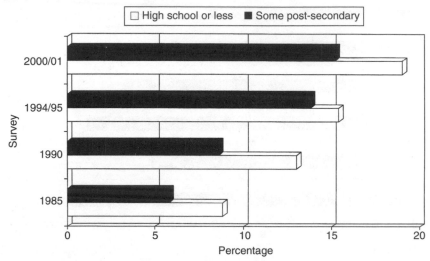

*Since BMI was collected only for a sub-sample composed of 20% of the 1978/79 CHS sample, the population estimates are unreliable and have been omitted.

Thus, an education effect is also observed for unhealthy exercise, an effect that is relatively consistent for all periods except 1990. Additionally, it appears that the improvement in exercise has been slightly greater for the higher-educated midlife population of Canada.

Obesity Rates and the Education Factor

Figure 9.3 presents the obesity rate (BMI 30+) for the low- and high-education groups and survey dates, except for the omission of the 1978/79 period, since only a small subset of individuals in the 1978/79 Canadian Health Survey were asked height and weight information. We observe that the education differential is again dramatic, especially when we compare the relative percentage difference in rates of obesity across the education groups (see Table A9.3, Appendix). In 1985, the obesity rate for midlife persons with post-secondary education is only 5.8% compared to 8.8% for persons with high school or less – a 3 percentage point difference, but a significant lower relative difference of 34%. In other words, persons with post-secondary education are about one-third less likely to be obese compared to those without post-secondary education in 1985. The education effect remains pervasive for the subsequent survey dates, but is relatively weak in 1994/95, and moderate in 2000/01. For this recent period (2000/01), it can be seen that the rate of obesity among the higher education group is 15.2% compared to 19% for the low-education category – a 20% lower rate in relative terms. A relative difference of 10.4% is observed for 1994/95. One can conclude that, while education is an important population health determinant of obesity, there may be some indications that the education effect is waning over time.

However, what is surprising is the fact that, although the obesity rates are higher among midlife persons with high school or less at all periods, the inflation in obesity has actually been greater in relative percentage terms for the high-education group between 1985 and 2000/01 than for the low-education group. For the low-education group, the obesity rate rose from 8.8% in 1985 to 19% in 2000/01 – a striking 116% rise over a period of only about 15 years. For the high-education cluster, the obesity rate jumped from 5.8% to 15.2% over the same period – an even more remarkable increase of 162% (see Table A9.3, Appendix).

Thus, obesity is also influenced by education level. Higher education is associated with healthy body weight. In addition, although the education effect appears to be softening in the 1990s, it is still moderately strong in 2000/01. But the most surprising finding is that the inflation in obesity rates between 1985 and 2000/01 has been almost 50% faster for the more educated group than for the lower one. This suggests that unhealthy diets and other behaviours linked to obesity have become the norm in society, and that the higher educated groups are catching up to their counterparts, although the gap remains about 20%.

Variable Patterns of Heavy Drinking across Education

As expected, the rate of heavy drinking among Canadians who are deemed to be in their midlife years (35–54) between 1978/79 and 2000/01 does not differ appreciably across education groups (see Figure 9.4). The one exception is for 1985, where it is observed that rates of heavy drinking are reported to be 9.6% among persons with post-secondary education and 6.3% for their counterparts. In contrast to the other health behaviours, persons with post-secondary education actually reported higher rates of heavy drinking than those without in four of the five survey dates. This pattern reverses for 2000/01, but again, the difference is borderline. Thus, the influence of education on rates of heavy drinking among midlife Canadians has remained weak, with indications of fluctuation, especially between 1985 and the adjacent periods as evidenced in Table A9.4 (Appendix).

Figure 9.4 Percentage of Canadian Population Aged 35–54 Who Are Heavy Drinkers* by Education Level, 1978/79–2000/01

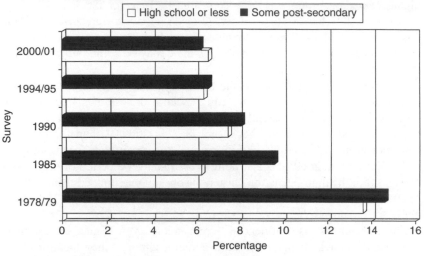

*Males = 14+ drinks/week; females = 12+ drinks/week.

Overall, the population health effect of increasing rates of educational attainment over time likely has had minimal impact on unhealthy drinking, since the education pattern is weak and inconsistent across the survey dates examined. More impressive, however, is the fact that there has been more than a 50% drop in heavy drinking rates since the late 70s for all midlife persons regardless of their education.

Income Differences in Baby Boomer Lifestyles: Are the Wealthier Healthier?

Let us turn to a similar analysis of lifestyle patterns across income levels for persons aged 35 to 54. We split income at the median level after converting into 2000 real dollars, which is necessary in order to make comparisons across time. It should be noted that this results in income splits that are not fifty-fifty, except for the most recent periods. The median income levels were approximated to be $14,000 for 1978/79; $23,000 for 1985; and $30,000 for 1990, 1994/95, 1998/99, and 2000/01. Although using income quintiles would result in more detailed and extreme comparisons of high and low income, we used only two categories to maintain low sampling variability and error. Also, this dichotomy will be relatively comparable to the dichotomous education variable used in the above analysis.

The Income Gradient of Smoking

Figure 9.5 exhibits smoking rates for midlife persons with low income and high income (above and below the median income for that period in 2000 dollars). It can be observed that persons aged 35 to 54 earning higher income have significantly lower rates of smoking for each of the survey years since 1978/79 (rates shown in Table A9.5, Appendix). The relative differences range between 18.1% and 39.9% lower. It is striking that this income effect appears to have become stronger over these decades, supporting research by Pappas et al. (1993). In 1978/79, smoking rates were 18.1% lower for midlife persons with higher incomes, but this differential strengthened to 39.9% lower in 2000/01. Thus, at the start of the new millennium, baby boomers over the median income are about one-third less likely to smoke than those under the median income. The actual prevalence rates in 2000/01 are 39.6% for lower-income baby boomers and only 23.8% for higher-income ones.

Figure 9.5 Percentage of Canadian Population Aged 35–54 Who Are Regular Smokers by Income Level*, 1978/79–2000/01

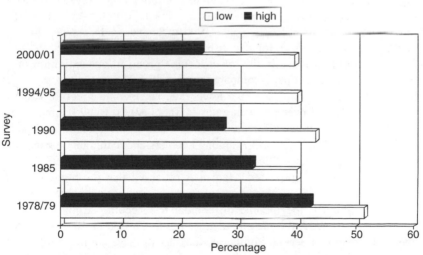

*Income levels are split at median based on 2000 real dollar conversions. The following median values were used: 1978/79 = \$14,000; 1985 = \$23,000; 1990, 1994/95, & 2000/01 = \$30,000.

This pattern is further delineated by comparing the within-group differences across the income categories and time period. The relative decrease in smoking between 1978/79 and 2000/01 is 23% (51.4% to 39.6%) for the lower-income group, but it is 43.5% (42.1% to 23.8%) for the higher-income group – a 19.5% differential. This confirms the magnification of the income effect over time by showing that the relative decline in smoking has occurred faster for midlife persons with higher incomes.

As discussed earlier, income in 2000 dollars rose about 24% between 1980 and 2000, but with most gains occurring in the 1980s. Thus, while income appears to exert a greater influence on smoking in the 1990s than in the previous decade in terms of income differentials, this 'income effect' likely has been further inflated by modest shifts in the income distribution mostly during the 1980s. It can be concluded that income is a strong determinant of smoking prevalence; and that the effect appears to be getting stronger; but that we have not fully capitalized on this pattern through improvements in real income in Canada over the last decade.

Unhealthy Exercise and Income

The percentage of the population aged 35 to 54 who are below the minimum exercise level (termed unhealthy exercise) by income group are shown in Figure 9.6 (also see Table A9.6, Appendix). Although the prevalence rate of unhealthy exercise is only slightly lower for persons with higher compared to lower income between 1978/79 and 1990 inclusive, there appears to be a developing income effect for exercise over the last few years. In 1994/95, 53.9% of midlife persons in the lower-income group fit our definition of an unhealthy exercise regiment, compared to only 48% of persons of similar age in the high-income group – a 10.9% lower rate. The income effect for 2000/01 results in a 21.2% lower rate (see rates in Table A9.6). Baby boomers with incomes below the median for the population had a 50.9% rate of unhealthy exercise compared to only 40.1% among boomers above that income cut-off.

The within-group rate of decline in unhealthy exercise between 1978/79 and 2000/01 can also be compared. Here it is observed that the higher-income group has enjoyed a 13.3% faster rate of decline in rates of unhealthy exercise. Therefore, although the income differential has become stronger between 1978/79 and 2000/01, the income distribution in Canada has only improved about 24% over that period. Similar to smoking, we have not made full use of this opportunity to make population-level improvements in exercise through this social determinant of health. However, it is noteworthy that rates of unhealthy exercise have declined appreciably for Canadians aged 35 to 54 between the late 1970s and the new century for both income groups. And

Figure 9.6 Percentage of Canadian Population Aged 35–54 Who Are Sedentary or Infrequent Exercisers* by Income Level**, 1978/79–2000/01

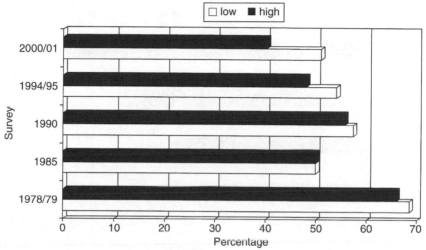

*15 min. of physical activity <3X per week.
**Income levels are split at median based on 2000 real dollar conversions. The following median values were used: 1978/70 = $14,000; 1985 = $23,000, 1990, 1994/95, & 2000/01 = $30,000.

finally, as observed in the earlier chapters, the decline in unhealthy exercise reversed temporarily sometime around the late 1980s or early 1990s.

Increasing Disparity in Obesity Rates by Income Level

The obesity rate (BMI 30+) for the low- and high-income groups is shown in Figure 9.7. While there has been a rise in the obesity rates for both income groups, it can be seen that the income effect has fluctuated between 1985 and 2000/01. The greatest differences between income groups occur in the 1990s. Although virtually no difference in obesity rates exists in 1985, we observe appreciable differences for the other survey periods, especially in the 1990s. The following are the relative percentage differences in rates between the low- and high-income groups of persons aged 35 to 54 in order of survey year: 2.5% (1985); –29.9% (1990); –18.1% (1994/95); and –9.8% (2000/01). Table A9.7 shows that in 1985, midlife persons in the low-income group had an obesity rate of 8%, whereas the high-income group reported 8.2%. These prevalence rates have risen significantly and differentially for midlife baby boomers in 2000/01 – to 18.3% (low-income group) and 16.5% (high-income group).

Figure 9.7 Percentage of Canadian Population Aged 35–54 Who Are Obese (BMI 30+) by Income Level*, 1985–2000/01**

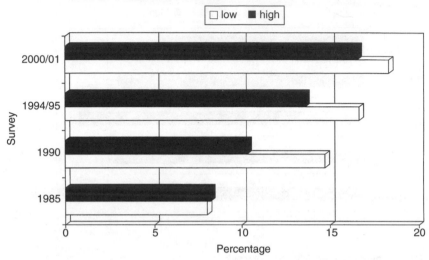

*Income levels are split at median based on 2000 real dollar conversions. The following median values were used: 1978/79 = $14,000; 1985 = $23,000; 1990, 1994/95, & 2000/01 = $30,000.
**Since BMI was collected only for a sub-sample composed of 20% of the 1978/79 CHS sample, the population estimates are unreliable and have been omitted.

It can also be observed that midlife persons in the lower half of the income distribution have experienced a 128.7% increase in the prevalence of obesity between 1985 and 2000/01, whereas the higher income had a 101.2% rise – a 27.5% difference between these two rates.

Thus, there is a moderate income effect for obesity, where we see that persons with higher income tend to have somewhat lower obesity rates in the population. Furthermore, the incline in obesity appears to have been somewhat more intense for midlife persons with lower incomes than for those with higher incomes, and there has been only minimal impact as the result of income-distribution shifts in the population to offset some of the increases in obesity.

Heavier Drinking among the Rich

Rates of heavy drinking have decreased substantially for midlife persons between 1978/79 and 2000/01, but not uniformly across income level. In

Figure 9.8 Percentage of Canadian Population Aged 35–54 Who Are Heavy Drinkers* by Income Level**, 1978/79–2000/01

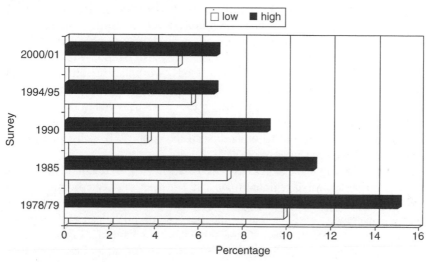

*Males = 14+ drinks/week; females = 12+ drinks/week.
**Income levels are split at median based on 2000 real dollar conversions. The following median values were used: 1978/79 = $14,000; 1985 = $23,000; 1990, 1994/95, & 2000/01 = $30,000.

addition, the influence of income on heavy drinking is considerably stronger than for the other lifestyle/health behaviours; however, it is in the opposite direction (see Table A9.8, Appendix). Rates of heavy drinking are consistently higher among those earning over the median-income level (also see Figure 9.8). The income effect has a range in relative percentage difference, between 17.5% and 145.9% higher, with the largest difference reported for 1990 and smaller differentials in the two more recent periods.

Additionally, the drop in the rate of heavy drinking between 1978/79 and 2000/01, which has occurred for both income groups, has been slightly (6.2%) larger for higher-income individuals (compare column percentages in Table A9.8, Appendix). Overall, rates of heavy drinking have fallen dramatically over these decades; they have decreased slightly faster for the higher-income group; and they also show a clear pattern of unhealthier drinking among the more rich, although the income effect appears to be waning since the peak in the 1990s.

The Regional Factor in Baby Boomer Lifestyles

Regional differences in health status and health behaviours are the result of a combination of individual and community-level factors, including socio-economic differences, employment opportunities, ethnic composition, culture, and even weather patterns. Regional differences also overlap with the social environment – communities, neighbourhoods, workplaces, and urban-rural composition (Yen and Syme, 1999). For instance, the higher unemployment rate and lower SES level of the Maritime provinces have led to poorer health outcomes in general. Additionally, Quebec's population is known for a proclivity to smoke. And, on the other side of the country, British Columbia is associated with higher rates of physical activity.

Health and lifestyle measures have been associated with region in numerous studies, but a definitive regional trend has not been uncovered. Quebec and British Columbia have been shown to have lower rates of obesity than the national average, an effect that is independent of birthplace (Cairney and Wade, 1999). However, Quebec and the Maritimes have the highest prevalence of smoking, and Quebec has a higher rate of sedentary behaviour than the rest of the country (Joffres and MacLean, 1999). The Maritime provinces, on the other hand, have had the highest rates of heavy drinking historically. Furthermore, mortality tends to be higher in census metropolitan areas (CMA) in the Atlantic provinces and Quebec, and lower in the Prairies and British Columbia (Gilmore and Gentleman, 1999). An analysis of changes in lifestyle behaviours between 1978/79 and 2000/01 may help to further elucidate these regional trends.

Regional Patterns in Smoking

Figure 9.9 presents smoking rates for midlife persons (aged 35–54) for the five regions under examination: Maritimes (Newfoundland, Prince Edward Island, Nova Scotia, New Brunswick), Quebec, Ontario, the Prairie provinces (Manitoba, Saskatchewan, and Alberta), and British Columbia. One should recall that smoking tends to peak around the midlife (35–54) years. Although the smoking rates have declined for all regions between 1978/79 and 2000/01, it has not been uniform. All regions, except for BC, have experienced a relative-percentage decline between 37% and 39% for the 22-year period. However, the decline for BC has been more pronounced – a striking 51.9% drop between 1978/79 and 2000/01 among persons aged 35 to 54. In addition, the prevalence of smoking for any given year across these regions is quite

Figure 9.9 Percentage of Canadian Population Aged 35–54 Who Are Regular Smokers by Region, 1978/79–2000/01

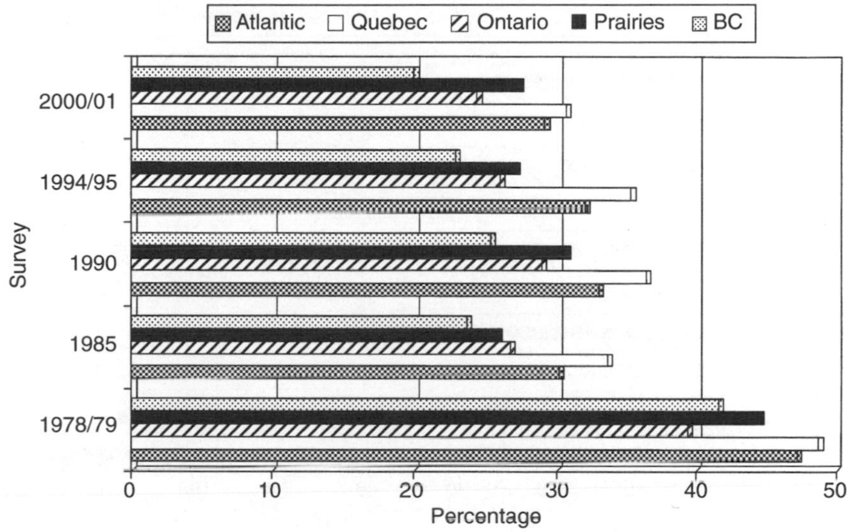

different. In 2000/01, the smoking rates among midlife baby boomers (i.e., persons in the 35–54 age group) were as follows: Quebec (30.6%); Maritimes (29.1%); Prairies (27.3%); Ontario (24.4%), and BC (20%). Thus, British Columbians clearly had the lowest smoking rates of the five regions in the most recent national health survey, in part because the decline in smoking over the last two decades has been the most dramatic for all regions (see these data in Table A9.9, Appendix).

An East-West Pattern to Unhealthy Exercise

The percentage of the midlife population exhibiting a sedentary or infrequent exercise level has also declined for all regions, as observed in Figure 9.10. The 22-year drop ranges from a 29% relative decrease for Quebec, and declines of 35.6% for Ontario, 40% for the Prairies, 42.9% for the Maritimes, and 45.5% for BC. Furthermore, the exercise level shows an east-west pattern. In 2000/ 01, rates of unhealthy exercise among baby boomers were as follows: Maritimes (43.9%); Quebec (47.8%); Ontario (41.6%); Prairies (40.8%); and BC (33.1%). Again, British Columbia stands in Canada with respect to physical activity indicators (see all of these rates in Table A9.10, Appendix).

Figure 9.10 Percentage of Canadian Population Aged 35–54 Who Are Sedentary or Infrequent Exercisers* by Region, 1978/79–2000/01

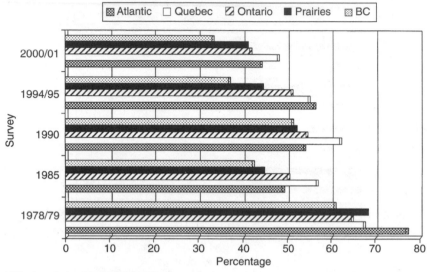

*15 min. of physical activity <3X per week.

Figure 9.11 Percentage of Canadian Population Aged 35–54 Who Are Obese (BMI 30+) by Region, 1985–2000/01

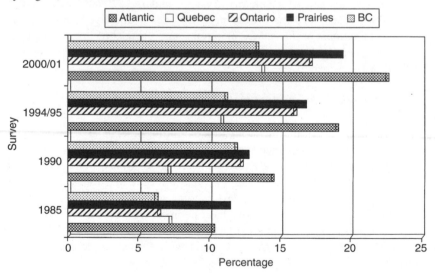

*Since BMI was collected only for a sub-sample composed of 20% of the 1978/79 CHS sample, the population estimates are unreliable and have been omitted.

Regional Differences in Obesity

Rates of obesity across the five regions reveal considerable diversity in terms of increases over time (only 1985–2000/01 data are available) and current levels among mid-life persons. The obesity rate (BMI 30+) has ballooned for all regions, as evidenced in Figure 9.11 (also see Table A9.11, Appendix). Between 1985 and 2000/01, it jumped 167% in Ontario; 120.5% in the Maritimes; 114% in BC; 90.3% in Quebec; and 70.7% in the Prairies. Thus, the increase in Ontario has been more than twice as high as for the Prairies. In 2000/01, we also observe a wide range in obesity among baby boomers (persons aged 35 to 54), with the Atlantic provinces exhibiting the highest rates, and BC and Quebec displaying the lowest rates. From high to low, the obesity prevalence rates are as follows: Atlantic (22.5%); Prairies (19.3%); Ontario (17.1%); Quebec (13.7%), and BC (13.3%).

Patterns of Heavy Drinking by Region

As presented in Figure 9.12, rates of heavy drinking have decreased substantially for midlife persons between 1978/79 and 2000/01, but not uniformly

Figure 9.12 Percentage of Canadian Population Aged 35–54 Who Are Heavy Drinkers* by Region, 1978/79–2000/01

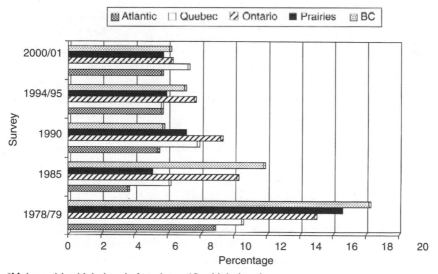

*Males = 14+ drinks/week; females = 12+ drinks/week.

across regions. Again, there appears to be an east-west trend in the decline over the 22-year period. The relative percentage decreases are as follows: a 36.4% decline in the Atlantic provinces; a 31.4% drop in Quebec; a 58.4% downturn in Ontario; a 66% decrease in the Prairies; and a 66.5% drop in BC. However, in 2000/01, the rate of heavy drinking is low in all regions, ranging between a low of 5.6% of the boomer population aged 35 to 54 living in the Atlantic and Prairie provinces, to a high of 7.2% for Quebec (see Table A9.12, Appendix).

In sum, it can be observed that there has been considerable regional variation in the prevalence of these four lifestyle indicators over time, as well as at a particular survey date. However, there is a general pattern: British Columbians are consistently the healthiest and those from the Atlantic Provinces are at the other extreme.

Foreign-Born Status and Baby Boomer Lifestyles

The analyses undertaken in the subsequent chapters have been based on baby boomers, who have been defined as persons born between 1946 and 1965. But our definition of a baby boom generation also entails a cultural component, one that distinguishes it from other generations. Thus, there is some controversy as to whether immigrants born outside of Canada constitute part of the baby boom generation, since they may not necessarily have embraced the liberal attitudes that characterize this generation. However, it is contended in this book that it is logical to include all Canadians in the baby boomer age cohorts because even foreign-born individuals will influence the future health and health care of our nation – a principal question guiding this research. It should be recalled that the research reviewed in Chapter 2 indicated that foreign-born persons tend to have better health when they come to Canada (the healthy immigrant effect), but lose that advantage over time. For these reasons, it is important to consider as well the potential effect of immigration on baby boomer health dynamics, especially since foreign-born status remains an important determinant of health in its own right (Toronto, 1993).

It has been estimated that 17.4% of the Canadian population is composed of foreign-born persons, what we term first-generation immigrants (Statistics Canada, 1998a). In 1978, 100,967 persons entered Canada, whereas in 2001, more than a quarter of a million (252,088) immigrants came (Statistics Canada, 2001a). The annual number of immigrants has therefore risen – from about 100,000 in the late 1970s and through the 1980s, to approximately 200,000 in the 1990s and early 2000s (see Chapter 2 for detailed trends). It has also been documented that the country of origin of immigrants has changed (Boyd and Vickers, 2000). Statistics Canada (1998a) data shows that immigrants originating from the United Kingdom and Europe declined from 90.3% prior to 1961, to about 19% between 1991 and 1996. In contrast, those coming from Asian and Middle Eastern countries have increased in proportion from 3% of all immigrants prior to 1961 to 57.1% between 1991 and 1996. We turn now to an analysis of the foreign-born effect on baby boomer lifestyles.

Foreign-Born Have Lower Smoking Rates

Smoking rates for midlife persons (aged 35–54) have been separated into foreign-born and Canadian-born groups in Figure 9.13 for four survey dates (1978/79 CHS, 1994/95 and 1998/99 NPHS, and 2000/01 CCHS). Note that foreign-born status was not collected in the 1985 and 1990 HPS. The striking decline in smoking can be observed in Figure 9.13 for both groups, but there are also some significant differences. Between 1978/79 and 2000/01, smoking declined from 35% to 15.6% for foreign-born persons (*a 55% decrease*), but only fell from 46.5% to 29.3% for Canadian-born persons (*a 37% drop*). It also can be ascertained that the foreign-born status gradient in smoking has increased, such that in 2000/01, Canadian-born are almost twice as likely to smoke as foreign-born. This positive influence on the smoking rate of midlife

Figure 9.13 Percentage of Canadian Population Aged 35–54 Who Are Regular Smokers by Foreign-Born Status, 1978/79–2000/01

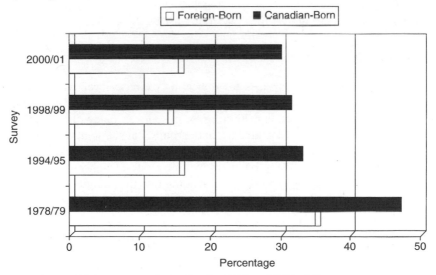

Note: Place of birth was not collected for the 1985 and 1990 HPS.

Figure 9.14 Percentage of Canadian Population Aged 35–54 Who Are Sedentary or Infrequent Exercisers* by Foreign-Born Status, 1978/79–2000/01

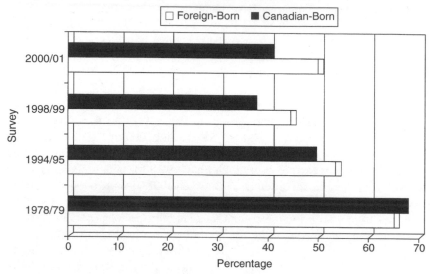

Note: Place of birth was not collected for the 1985 and 1990 HPS.
*15 min. of physical activity <3X per week.

Canadians is magnified by the fact that the foreign-born proportion of the population is increasing over time (see Table A9.13, Appendix).

Higher Unhealthy Exercise Levels among Foreign-Born

A very different picture surfaces for unhealthy exercise level, as shown in Figure 9.14. Canadian-born are the ones with the advantage. Also, the percentage of the mid-life population exhibiting exercise levels below the minimum recommended amount has declined for both groups, but at a somewhat steeper rate for Canadian-born (see rates in Table A9.14, Appendix). For example, in 2000/01, Canadian-born baby boomers exhibit a rate of unhealthy exercise that is fully 10 percentage points lower than the rate for foreign-born (39.9% compared to 49.9%).

Foreign-Born Are Less Obese

Rates of obesity across the foreign-born status variable are only available between 1994/95 and 2000/01, as can be seen in Figure 9.15. Between these

Figure 9.15 Percentage of Canadian Population Aged 35–54 Who Are Obese (BMI 30+) by Foreign-Born Status, 1994/95–2000/01

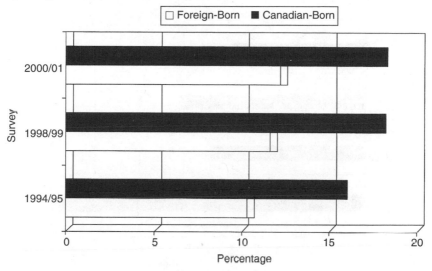

Note: Place of birth was not collected for the 1985 and 1990 HPS.
*Since BMI was collected only for a sub-sample composed of 20% of the 1978/79 CHS sample, the population estimates are unreliable and have been omitted.

dates, the obesity rate (BMI 30+) has risen from 10.3% to 12.2% among the foreign-born, but from 15.6% to 17.9% among the Canadian-born (shown in Table A9.15, Appendix). Thus, the obesity rate is about *one-third lower* for foreign-born persons of baby boom ages. However, both groups have experienced approximately the same incline in the rate of obesity over this relatively short period of six years (see Figure 9.15). Therefore, it would appear that, while the foreign-born experience some advantage over the Canadian-born midlife population in terms of unhealthy body weight, both groups are following a similar upward trajectory.

Patterns of Heavy Drinking by Foreign-Born Status

As presented in Figure 9.16, rates of heavy drinking have decreased substantially for midlife persons between 1978/79 and 2000/01, but at a faster rate among foreign-born individuals. Between 1978/79 and 2000/01, the percentage of heavy drinkers dwindled from 13.5% to only 3.3% among the foreign-born (see Table A9.16, Appendix). For the Canadian-born, the rate dropped

Figure 9.16 Percentage of Canadian Population Aged 35–54 Who Are Heavy Drinkers*
by Foreign-Born Status, 1978/79–2000/01

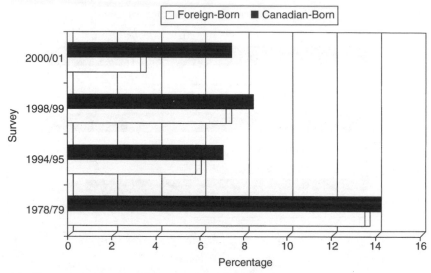

Note: Place of birth was not collected for the 1985 and 1990 HPS.
*Males = 14+ drinks/week; females = 12+ drinks/week.

from 14% to 7.2%. As seen in Figure 9.16, heavy drinking among foreign-born
persons of baby boomer age in 2000/01 is *less than half* the rate observed for
Canadian-born boomers. However, the rate of heavy drinking has clearly
shown tremendous improvement over the 22-year span.

10

Summarizing Population and Baby Boomer Health Dynamics

The Big Picture

We started this journey by asking questions about how the baby boomers are aging, and, the broader question, how lifestyles are developed, sustained, and changed as we age. The Social Change Model forms the theoretical backbone of the analyses conducted in this book. This model offers a dynamic method to the understanding of the interconnections of individual and structural factors by means of amalgamating elements of age stratification, life course, and cohort approaches to the study of aging. A fundamental axiom at the core of this perspective is that population health is moulded and remoulded as successive cohorts move through their life cycle as if on an upward-bound escalator. The incline of the escalator can be conceived as representing various health characteristics, such as the prevalence of healthy lifestyles or chronic illnesses, and which constantly readjust according to the complex interplay of macro (structural), meso (policy), and micro (individual) changes tied to cohorts and individuals. This led to a brief review of other advancements in healthy lifestyle theories.

The baby boom generation is central to this conceptualization because of its size and placement within the age structure. Using our 20-year definition entailing persons born between 1946 and 1965, who would have been aged 36 to 55 in 2001, it can be observed from Canadian Census data that there were 9,405,055 baby boomers out of a total population of 30,007,095 in 2001. This generation comprised a remarkable 31.3% of the Canadian population. The front edge of this bulge in the age structure will turn 65 in 2011, 75 in 2021, and 85 in 2031, at which point all baby boomers will have reached their elder years (65+). Without a doubt, of any generation the baby boomers have and will continue to have the single greatest influence on social, economic, and health patterns, the latter of which will become magnified as baby boomers move along the life course trajectory. Yet, to assume that these individuals are homogeneous, or that their impact on society will be unidimensional, over-looks the complexity facing us. Moreover, elaboration of baby boomer health dynamics necessitates examination of age, period, and cohort patterns, and this in turn requires placing these age groups and cohorts into the context of patterns for the total population, across time, and for key determinants of health. For this reason, while the focus of this research has been on baby boomers, the health dynamics of the total population of Canadians is of paramount importance. We have also discovered that many of the same shifts in healthy lifestyles noted for baby boomers appear to have filtered throughout the total population. We now attempt to highlight and synthesize some of the major health trends based on what has been ascertained in the previous chapters. Discussion of the implications of patterns will follow in a subsequent chapter.

Population and Baby Boomer Smoking: Putting Out the Fire

One of the most significant changes in healthy lifestyles over the last couple of decades has been the decline in rates of smoking for men and women. It is estimated in this study that, for the total male population aged 15 and over, the prevalence of smoking has dropped sharply, from 43.9% in 1978/79 (CHS) to 24.6% in 2001/01 (CCHS). For females, smoking prevalence has decreased from 35.8% in 1978/79 to 20.2% in 2000/01. Although the rate of female teenage smoking (using those aged 15–19) surfaced as a problem in the 1990s, showing an escalation from 19% in 1990 (HPS) to 20.9% in 1994/95 (NPHS), and peaking at 25.2% in 1998/99 (NPHS), the rate has actually dropped in 2000/01 to 18.8%. And while about one in five teenage young women smoke in 2000/01, there is not much of a rise in the smoking rate for young adult or middle-aged women. Indeed, the inverted U-shaped curve for smoking rates across the ages for women has flattened considerably. Additionally, women in their childbearing years have exhibited some of the most dramatic declines in smoking rates. For example, those aged 25 to 29 in 2000/01 had a rate of 22% compared to 32.7% only six years earlier, in 1994/95. Furthermore, there seems to be some degree of slowing in the decline in smoking when we follow the trajectories of specific cohorts. This may signify the need for more aggres-sive targeted health promotion strategies to make further improvements. With respect to gender differences in smoking, there has been a steady decline in the male/female smoking gap between 1978/79 and 2000/01, potentially reflect-ing an end to the gendered nature of cigarette smoking.

Turning to the baby boomers, rates of smoking are 40.4% lower among baby boomers (persons aged 35–54 in 2000/01) than persons this age in 1978/79, approximately a generation apart. Also noteworthy is the fact that the greatest downturn in smoking rates for the baby boomers, as well as for other cohorts for that matter, appears to have taken place between 1978/79 and 1985. Whether this is indicative of historical events occurring during those years, or whether it has become increasingly difficult to recruit quitters from the shrinking pool of diehard smokers, is difficult to ascertain from these data. Overall, there has been a steady downward trend in smoking rates between the late 1970s and the start of the new millennium that has permeated virtually all age and sex groups in Canadian society.

Population and Baby Boomer Unhealthy Exercise Levels:
Room for Improvement

Consistent with our focus on lifestyle behaviours associated with illness risk, patterns of unhealthy exercise levels were also investigated. This measure includes persons reporting exercise levels that are below recommended guidelines; that is, less than three exercise intervals a week of at least 15 to 20 minutes in duration each. The type of activity examples provided in the surveys includes brisk walking, jogging, racket sports, weight training, and various other aerobic exercises. Although more sophisticated measures, such as physical activity or exercise energy, or metabolic expenditure, are available in recent surveys, the data needed to create them was not collected prior to the mid-1990s. The more crude measure used in this research still provides a very useful indicator of physical activity.

Contrary to many portrayals in the media, the proportion of Canadians engaging in unhealthy exercise has fallen 28% for males and 34% for females between the late 1970s and the beginning of this century. Furthermore, the 10% gender gap in exercise levels that favoured men at just about every age group has vanished, except for females aged 15 to19 and elderly women aged 70 and over. Also noteworthy is the fact that a significant proportion of the gains in exercise between the late 1970s and the mid-1980s were lost some time during the late 1980s and early 1990s. In fact, the 1994/95 rates of unhealthy exercise were no better than what was observed in 1985, with 1990 showing a clear reversal in the period trend. The two groups that have experienced the most dramatic reversal in the late 1980s are females aged 15 to19 and middle-aged males.

The decline in unhealthy exercise was even more pronounced among the baby boomers in 2000/01 compared to persons their age in 1978/79. This rate fell 40.9%, which can be compared to the 31% decline for the total population aged 15 and over. Thus, the boomers have led the way in terms of making relative gains over the 22-year period, regardless of whether they were younger or older boomers. However, while boomers, as well as Canadians of all ages, are embracing an active lifestyle to a greater extent today, there is considerable room for improvement. Approximately 40% of Canadians of any age are deemed to be in the unhealthy exercise range; and approximately two out of three are not reaping the full benefits of an active lifestyle, a pattern that is nothing short of a national tragedy from a population health perspective.

Population and Baby Boomer Obesity: A Bulging Bulge

We also analysed patterns of the population who report a body mass index (BMI) of 30 and over. This is considered to be at the high end of obesity definitions, but serves this analysis well. This more conservative measure better correlates with body fat, and, moreover, it is a stronger risk factor for diabetes, cardiovascular disease, and arthritis. We began with the year 1985, since the 1978/79 CHS only asked this question of a subset of individuals that could not be used for subgroups. Yet, even studying the period between 1985 and 2000/01, we can clearly observe a shocking trend – a *doubling* of the obesity rate for men and women. For males aged 20 to 64, the prevalence of obesity has jumped from 7.1% in 1985 to 16.3% in 2000/01; and for females of similar age the rate has *nearly tripled*, from 5.8% to 14.2%. Additionally, this bulging obesity rate has shown an almost perfect upward linear trajectory over these years. The pattern of obesity across the life span has also taken new shape. There has been a sharper incline in the obesity rate among people in their 20s than in the past, when the rise typically occurred at midlife. Evidence that we have become a heavier nation as a whole is evidenced in the average BMI figures, which show that mean BMI levels have moved from the accept-able range (18.5–24.9) into the overweight range (25–29.9) between 1985 and 2000/01. Specifically, for the male population aged 20 to 64, the average BMI increased from 24.81 in 1985 to 26.24 in 2000/01; for females, it rose from 23.30 to 24.83.

The obesity rate for baby boomers in 2000/01 (using persons aged 35–54) is 16.2%, compared to about half that rate (8.2%) in 1985 among persons of that age. Not surprisingly, obesity rates have risen faster among the younger baby boomers (persons aged 35–44 in 2000/01) than the older ones (persons aged 45–54 in 2000/01). Moreover, the spread of obesity has been so pervasive that virtually every age and sex group in the population has been affected. But the fact that the aging pattern of obesity has taken a different shape, one that now encompasses young people, has serious and far-reaching health consequences for Canadian society. These findings parallel those that have also shown dramatic inclines in obesity among children.

Population and Baby Boomer Heavy Drinking: Three Cheers

In this research, we used 14 or more drinks a week for men and 12 or more for women as our threshold for heavy drinking, given gender differences in body mass. Rates of heavy drinking have dropped by more than half for the adult Canadian population, but a wide gender gap persists. For males aged 15 and over, the percentage reporting heavy drinking declined from 21.8% in 1978/79 to 10.1% in 2000/01, whereas for females the drop was from 7% in 1978/79 to 3.1% in 2000/01. The largest erosion in rates of heavy drinking has occurred between 1978/79 and 1985, indicating that the late 1970s marked the end of an era when surfeit drinking was considered to be acceptable or at least tolerated. Also, the reduction in heavy drinking has been more intensive for certain groups – for example, males aged 20 to 29 and females aged 15 to 39, but the gender differential remains the most dominant pattern.

It is not surprising, therefore, that we also have found that baby boomers drink considerably less than their counterparts a generation earlier. In 2000/01, 6.3% of persons aged 35 to 54 (comprising 95% of the baby boomers) reported heavy drinking compared to 13.8% in 1978/79, a rate of heavy drinking that is half as large as the generation two decades earlier. Also, it has been shown that the greatest decline appears to be between the late 1970s and 1985 for the 22-year period under study, and has occurred in much the same manner for older and younger baby boomers.

Population and Baby Boomer Health Status: Ups and Downs

Analyses of chronic illness as well as doctor visits, for the total population and for baby boomers, revealed a number of contradictory patterns. The measure of chronic conditions is a broad-based variable that includes conditions such as asthma, arthritis, diabetes, hypertension, heart problems, and so on. Between 1978/79 and 2000/01, there has been about a 29% increase in the prevalence of chronic conditions among males aged 15 and over, and about a 20% rise for females of the same age, with most of the period increase occurring among persons under the age of 50. However, the most pronounced aging pattern is the sharp rise in the chronic illness rate after age 50, especially among the elderly, as might be expected. This has not changed appreciably over the time period under study. Additionally, it appears that the rate of chronic illness has risen faster in the 1990s. The baby boomers as a whole follow these same trends; for instance, baby boomers aged 35 to 54 in 2000/01 have a 19% higher rate of chronic conditions than persons of the same age in 1978/79. However, younger baby boomers have shown a greater increase in chronic conditions compared to persons their age in 1978/79, and to older boomers (29% and 11.3%, respectively). This is consistent with the population trend showing that the most significant rise in chronic illness over time has occurred among persons under the age of 50. Whether this is an indication of poorer health over time for these individuals or whether it reflects more sensitive diagnostic methods for detecting chronic illness is left for future study.

This measure combines any chronic condition; thus it is important also to examine specific ones. But since the prevalence of these individual conditions is relatively low in the younger ages, we start with age 45 for the population analysis. A major risk factor for cardiovascular disease, hypertension rates have risen sharply. Between 1978/79 and 2000/01, the hypertension rate for men aged 45 and over jumped from 15% to 24% (a 60% increase). For women, the rate only rose from 24.6% to 27.9% (a 13% increase), but the hypertension rate is actually higher for women than it is for men as noticed in the prevalence rates. Also, the rate moves sharply upward in the elder years for both men and women, indicating strong aging effects, although ones that are not necessarily becoming magnified with time.

Baby boomers aged 35 to 54 in 2000/01 have reported a hypertension rate of 9.7% compared to 8.1% among persons that age in 1978/79, or a 19.7% higher rate. As with chronic conditions, the rate of hypertension has actually risen more among younger baby boomers (a 47.5% increase compared to persons 35–44 in 1978/79) than for older boomers (only an 11.8% increase). This pattern is also consistent with our lifestyle pattern, telling us that the younger boomers have not made the same gains as older boomers in terms of smoking declines, and have faired worse in terms of obesity rates, which are correlated with hypertension.

We also investigated the prevalence of arthritis, but found little significant change. The arthritis rate for men aged 40 and over has hovered between 20% and 21% for the period 1978/79 to 2000/01. For women of this age, the rate has also remained stable over this period, but at a higher level. Arthritis is between 1.5 and 2 times higher among women than among men. Also, as expected, the arthritis rate swings upward sharply with age. Furthermore, baby boomers aged 35 to 54 in 2000/01 have actually experienced a small (7.3%) drop in arthritis compared to persons this age in 1978/79.

Turning to diabetes, we observe a more alarming pattern. The diabetes rate for men aged 45 and over has more than doubled in 22 years, from 4.1% in

1978/79 to 9.8% in 2000/01. A similar but less intense trend has occurred for women aged 45 and over, a rise from 4.6% to 7.4% between 1978/79 and 2000/01. The diabetes rate has increased the fastest among middle-aged men and women, and mirror patterns of obesity presented above. In addition, baby boomers in 2000/01 have experienced 76.5% inflation in their diabetes rate compared with persons their age in 1978/79. And the accelerating rate of diabetes has permeated both younger and older boomers alike.

We have also witnessed an upturn in doctor visits. There has been a 60.2% rise between 1978/79 and 2000/01 in the number of males aged 15 and over reporting three or more doctor visits in the prior year. Females have exhibited a 40.5% incline in three or more doctor visits in a year over that same period. Also, for both genders, the propensity to visit a doctor shows a fairly strong upswing after age 50, and peaks in the older ages as expected. However, it is noteworthy that while most age groups have experienced relatively similar increases over the 22-year span, the 15 to 19 age group has stood out – where teenage males had a doubling (97% rise) in the rate and teenage females exhibited a 85% increase. Furthermore, it can be observed in our most recent data (2000/01 CCHS) that females begin with considerably higher rates of doctor visits than males, and that these differences remain across the life cycle, but eventually converge among the elderly, resulting in a about a one-third higher rate overall. Gender differences associated with the period of life devoted to childbearing only accounts for part of this gap.

Baby boomers are not immune to the incline in rates for doctor visits. Between 1978/79 and 2000/01, there was a 48.6% increase in this rate when comparing persons of baby boomer age in 2000/01 with their age counterparts in the earlier time period. This more frequent medical attention has occurred for both the younger and older baby boomers equally. The greater attention of the health care system devoted to baby boomers aged 35 to 54 in 2000/01 may be indicative of things to come.

The data pertaining to doctor visits point to movement towards increased medicalization of the population at all ages. As expected, the elderly are receiving the greatest intensity of health care. These analyses are consistent with other literature demonstrating a continued rise in health care spending per capita, particularly physician billings and pharmaceutical costs, especially for older persons (see, especially, Evans et al., 2001). Regardless, it is difficult to ascertain the exact number of doctor visits associated with maximum health benefit.

Socio-economic, Regional, and Foreign-Born Status Factors

Baby boomer health dynamics were also detailed by comparing across high and low categories of education and income for persons aged 35 to 54 at the various survey dates. The education dichotomy was defined as high school or less, compared with at least some post-secondary education, whereas we used above and below the median income in real dollars for the second analysis. In addition, patterns are elucidated across five major regions in Canada, and by foreign-born status. Note that midlife Canadians are the baby boomers in 2000/01. We turn first to the influence of education on the lifestyles of baby boomers.

The 'Education Effect' in Baby Boomer Healthy Lifestyles

Taken together, there has been a relatively strong education effect for smoking and obesity rates for midlife persons aged 35 to 54, who approximate the baby boomers in 2000/01. Those with post-secondary education exhibited lower rates of these lifestyle factors when comparing them against the surveys dates under examination. The education effect on unhealthy exercise levels has been less striking, but persistent. Heavy drinking does not seem to be influenced a great deal by education level, and thus revealed fluctuations in the patterns. It is possible that the curvilinear association between SES and drinking masks differences in this health behaviour.

The relative change in unhealthy lifestyles over the survey years has also been different for the two educational groups, and, moreover, suggests very different patterns for the four lifestyles. The drop in smoking and heavy drinking has been slightly more pronounced for midlife Canadians with post-secondary education, whereas the opposite pattern has been discovered for unhealthy exercise. But even this difference is only borderline. The most salient difference is observed for changes in obesity rates. The lower-educated group actually experienced a smaller rise in obesity than those with post-secondary education – about a 50% differential. Thus, it would appear that the spread of unhealthy body mass has become so prevalent that it is cutting across all education gradients. Simply, midlife Canadians with higher education have been fast approaching the obesity levels of their counterparts, and have only about a 20% differential left to consume.

The 'Income Effect' in Baby Boomer Healthy Lifestyles

Using a median income cut-off after adjusting for inflation, it has been shown that having a higher income level moderately decreases the rate of smoking and unhealthy exercise; it has a modest effect in the same direction for the prevalence of obesity, but has a stronger but opposite effect for rates of heavy drinking. These trends are remarkably similar to the ones uncovered for the education differential, especially for the baby boomer analysis, except that midlife persons with higher income tend to drink more heavily than lower-income persons (compared to the education differential in drinking patterns). However, what stands out is that both the income and the education effects have not always been uniform over time. Taking obesity as an example, it has been demonstrated that while obesity has been on the increase for all midlife groups between 1985 and 2000/01 in Canada, and tends to be spreading faster among both low-educated and low-income groups at any particular time period, there are interesting nuances. The obesity rate has been rising consider-ably faster for midlife persons with post-secondary education than those with-out, whereas it is the lower-income persons who have been increasing their obesity at a faster rate, although the rate change is very small.

Unlike education, real median income has only risen by about 24% between 1980 and 2001, and most of this change occurred during the 1980s. If relative income levels do in fact increase to a greater extent in the future, then the income effect likely will have more positive population health consequence for these particular health lifestyle behaviours, except in the case of heavy drinking, because here higher income has an opposite effect. However, there are indications that the income effect for healthy lifestyles has not lost its influence over the last two decades, and, indeed, that it may be intensifying for smoking and the prevalence of unhealthy exercise. Conversely, the obesity and heavy drinking patterns over time suggest some weakening of the income effect. Overall, income persists in being an important determinant of lifestyle health behaviours and population health; however, recently we have been more successful in improving the education level of Canadians than we have in raising relative income levels. Regardless, the socio-economic status factor continues to be a primary determinant of health as well as for healthy lifestyles.

The 'Regional Effect' in Baby Boomer Healthy Lifestyles

The five regions used to study health dynamics include the Maritimes (New-foundland, Prince Edward Island, Nova Scotia, New Brunswick), Quebec, Ontario, the Prairie provinces (Manitoba, Saskatchewan, and Alberta), and British Columbia. Except for BC, all regions have experienced a relative percentage decline in smoking between 37% and 39% for the 22-year period. However, the decrease for BC boomers compared to the previous generation has been 51.9%. Additionally, the prevalence of smoking among baby boomers in 2000/01 is highest in Quebec and lowest in BC: Quebec (30.6%); Maritimes (29.1%); Prairies (27.3%); Ontario (24.4%), and BC (20%). All regions have also experienced significant decreases in sedentary or infrequent exercise, ranging between a 29% decline for Quebec and a 45.5% for BC. The recent (2000/01) trends in unhealthy exercise reveal an east-west pattern, from a high of 43.9% in the Maritimes to a low of 33.1% in BC. However, obesity rates across the five regions uncover a different picture. Between 1985 and 2000/01, they jumped 167% in Ontario, 120.5% in the Maritimes, 114% in BC, 90.3% in Quebec, and 70.7% in the Prairies. In 2000/01, obesity among baby boomers is highest in the Maritimes, whereas BC and Quebec have the lowest rates. Rates of heavy drinking have decreased substantially for midlife persons between 1978/79 and 2000/01, again with an east-west trend in the decline over the 22-year period. And in 2000/01, the rate of heavy drinking has remained low in all regions.

Overall, considerable regional diversity exists in the prevalence of these four lifestyle indicators, both over time and today. The singular pattern that is repeated, however, has been that British Columbians are the healthiest and those from the Atlantic provinces are at the other extreme for virtually all unhealthy lifestyles that we have studied.

The 'Foreign-Born Status Effect' in Baby Boomer Healthy Lifestyles

Foreign-born persons of baby boomer age in 2000/01 were considerably better off in terms of smoking, obesity, and heavy drinking than were Canadian-born persons. Conversely, the latter enjoyed an advantage with respect to exercise level. For example, foreign-born persons aged 35 to 54 in 2000/01 were half as likely to smoke, less than half as likely to drink heavily, and approximately one-third less likely to be obese, whereas Canadian-born boomers exhibited a rate of unhealthy exercise that is about 20% lower in relative terms than the foreign-born.

Taken together, it would appear that the lifestyle portrait of the baby boomers has been significantly improved through immigration over time. Foreign-born persons probably are in better health and exhibit better lifestyle behaviours than the Canadian-born population for several reasons. First, there is a strong selection effect. Second, the countries of origin have shifted more to Asian and Southern Asian countries, whose populations seem to exhibit healthier lifestyle behaviours. The one exception pertains to exercise levels, which is not to say that the 40% rate of unhealthy exercise among the Canadian-born is acceptable, but that it is significantly better than the 50% level found among foreign-born persons of baby boomer age. Overall, even though the foreign-born comprise about 17% of the Canadian population, they still reflect a healthy lifestyle immigrant effect that improves population health in terms of smoking, obesity, and heavy drinking.

11

Explicating Two Lifestyle-Health Paradoxes

Our study of baby boomers, as well as the full Canadian population, has revealed a number of complex health trends. Although we have observed considerable variation across age cohorts, gender, socio-economic status, region, foreign-born status, and time period, several definitive patterns have surfaced. There has been a substantially lower rate of smoking, unhealthy exercise, and heavy drinking between the late 1970s and the early 2000s. Concomitantly, there has been an unprecedented sharp rise in obesity. Additionally, we have witnessed a modest incline in the total number of chronic conditions over this time period with particularly dramatic increases in diabetes. Doctor visits have risen between 1978/79 and 2000/01, but appear to have reached a threshold since the mid-1990s. These trends in health dynamics suggest that there are a number of health conundrums for which explanations are not readily apparent, and which therefore beckon deeper probing into prominent shifts in the social and behavioural fabric of Canadian society.

The Exercise-Obesity Paradox

There is a paradox embedded within the concurrent trends of decreasing levels of unhealthy exercise and a significant rise in unhealthy body weight over the last few decades. In order to explain these discordant patterns, changes in leisure-time physical activity, television watching, work-related activity, eating habits, and environmental factors influencing healthy lifestyles will be examined.

Are the Patterns for Leisure-Time Physical Activity Similar?

We have established that there has been a sizable decline in the percentage of the Canadian population, including the baby boomers, reporting levels of exercise that do not meet minimum recommendations, what we term un-healthy exercise. However, these data were based on questions pertaining to frequency of engaging in exercise of a particular type, intensity, and duration that may not tap into all levels of physical activity. It is necessary therefore to consider leisure-time and work-related physical activity as well. Leisure-time physical activity is measured by assessing total energy expenditure in kilocalo-ries (kcal) burned per kilogram (kg) per day. Physical inactivity has been typically measured as expending less than 3 kcal/kg/day, or approximately 200 kcal, which is equivalent to about 30 minutes of brisk walking (Katzmarzyk, 2001). This measure may include more activities than one simply based on a survey question amalgamating frequency and a minimum duration of exercise. However, one would expect that they overlap significantly. A review of all available studies that have conducted comparative analyses of national health surveys indicates that there has been a significant upturn in leisure-time physical activity between 1981 and 2000, and, conversely, a decrease in the prevalence of inactivity (Canadian Population Health Initiative, 2004; Curtis, White, and McPherson, 2000; Federal, Provincial and Territorial Advisory Committee on Population Health, 1999; Statistics Canada, 1999c; Physical Activity Monitor, 2000). Thus, it would appear that parallel trends have occurred for leisure-time physical activity and the exercise measure used in the present study, leaving the exercise-obesity paradox unexplained.

Is Television the Culprit?

Many people believe that television watching has become a national pastime to the extent that active lifestyles are compromised, and, furthermore, that this leisure-time pursuit leads to unhealthy body weight among a significant pro-portion of our population. Additionally, this health hazard has been viewed as particularly problematic among children and teenagers. Undoubtedly, the ex-pansion of cable and digital television, and television connections to satellite, VCRs, and DVDs, have escalated the availability of home entertainment. The question is whether this availability has resulted in significantly longer hours of watching television, and whether this in turn has translated into lengthened sedentary behaviour and subsequent increases in obesity rates over the period of study.

    Like other research, analysing the relationship between television watching and body weight is complex and fraught with issues associated with establish-ing a causal association. Central to this issue is demonstrating that a particular lifestyle behaviour precedes, as well as influences, a specific outcome. Gener-ally, research studies corroborate a positive association between television watching and obesity, although a few studies have been inconclusive (Jeffery and French, 1998; Tucker and Bagwell, 1991; Tucker and Friedman, 1989). Most research is based on children, and these studies tend to use cross-sectional data – that is, data collected at one point in time. The first problem limits our ability to generalize to adults, whereas the second limits the ability to draw inferences of *causal* evidence. Unless a prospective or longitudinal approach is used, a correlation between television watching and obesity could mean several things. It could simply reflect the fact that obese individuals watch more television because they are generally more sedentary, rather than the opposite. Alternatively, it could provide evidence that television watching does indeed magnify the probability of being obese.

One authoritative study in this area is presented in a recent article by Jeffery and French (1998), in which they followed 198 men (combined income group), 529 high-income women, and 332 low-income women between the ages of 20 and 45 over a one-year period. In this research, the relationships among television viewing, fast food eating, and body mass index were examined using cross-sectional data as well as panel data spanning a one-year period. The researchers also controlled for the potentially confounding effects of several socio-demographic and health variables deemed to be additional determinants of this health outcome (e.g., age, education, smoking status). Interestingly, Jeffery and French discovered that time in front of a television and fast food meals are both associated with obesity for women, and especially their sub-sample of low-income women, and at the cross-sectional level of analysis. However, their research does not support a similar association for men. Moreover, at the longitudinal level of analysis, only a marginal, weak association (one that approaches but does not meet scientific standards of statistical significance) between television watching and body mass index is found for high-income women, but not for any other groups. In addition, they did not obtain statistical support for a correlation between television watching and level of exercise for any group, an association that one would expect to uncover if in fact television compromised active leisure-time pursuits. Thus, we are left wondering whether the portrayal of North Americans glued to the television and becoming couch potatoes is true, and whether television is the culprit where North Americans becoming inactive and overweight is concerned. This appears to go against the more positive image portrayed by statistical trends in exercise and leisure-time physical activity.

Certainly there is an intuitive appeal to the television-inactivity-obesity relationship, and, indeed, there may be a modest relationship between television watching and obesity. But we require more evidence before we can conclude that the 'obesity epidemic' is due to television watching per se, as espoused (ironically) by the popular psychologist Dr Phil on numerous television shows. Partial evidence can be obtained at the population-level if we were to establish that there have been heightened rates of television watching that precede or coincide with the elevation in rates of obesity. Of course, even if population trends in television viewing shift in one direction, it does not necessarily mean that all persons or subgroups in that population have followed suit. Yet, if the population health changes are significant, in all probability they would filter through substantial segments of society.

To begin, we know that obesity rates have risen during the 1980s, and especially the 1990s. It is interesting, however, that data on television watching actually reveal that the average weekly viewing time has decreased or remained approximately the same between the mid-1980s and today. For example, data show that a drop has occurred in the average length of time Canadians sit in front of a television – from 23.3 hours in 1991 to 21.5 hours in 2000 (Statistics Canada, 2001). Furthermore, in 2000, the lowest rate (13.2 hours per week) was reported for young men aged 18 to 24; and teens and children reported only 14.1 hours and 15.5 hours per week, respectively. Adult women actually reported the highest levels, at 25.5 hours per week. Taken together, the available evidence suggests that while television viewing and obesity may be correlated, and perhaps causally connected for certain groups at an attenuated level, time in front of a television set does not appear to have risen substantially, at least during the 1990s. Thus, we are not drawn to the conclusion that television is the main or only culprit in the proliferation of unhealthy body weight, nor is it responsible for a significant proportion of the population falling below the recommended activity guidelines.

Is Work-Related Physical Activity the Problem for Adults?

Turning to work activity, it is possible that the increasingly technologically driven market has created more sedentary work time. One indicator of this is computer use patterns. Data from the General Social Survey (Statistics Canada, 2001b) shows that computer use in jobs has almost doubled over the last decade—from 33% in 1989 to 57% in 2000. And the vast majority of Canadians (80%) work at their computer every day, at work or at home. But even if some manual labour jobs have become more sedentary because of computerization and the integration of advanced technology, for many white-collar jobs the computer has only replaced the typewriter or other activities conducted at a desk. We also have not observed a definitive upward pattern in rates of unhealthy exercise across education or income groups, as shown in Chapter 9. In fact, the associations between exercise and socio-economic status were modest, about a 20% differential. A moderate or strong relationship would have provided at least indirect evidence in support of work-related causes of inactivity. It therefore is doubtful that, if indeed there has been a trend towards more sedentary work behaviour, it has been significant enough to counter the overall rise in reported exercise and leisure-time physical activity levels presented for all age and sex groups in earlier chapters.

Thus, overall, exercise and leisure-time physical measures tell the same story: people have become less sedentary, and, conversely, more active since the late 1970s. It is possible that some of this improvement may be lost during work hours, given that we have become more of a high-tech, work station-based workforce, but the weight of this factor is not enough to tip the scales. Moreover, television watching does not appear to be a significant factor in the transformation of exercise patterns and may be only weakly associated with obesity. The same logic can be applied to computer use at home. A synthesis of these trends indicates that it does not appear that Canadians have become more sedentary in their lifestyles since the 1970s, even though unhealthy physical activity levels in our population are too high. In other words, the improvements in activity levels observed since the late 1970s have not been significant enough in and of themselves to offset other unhealthy behaviours associated with obesity. In addition, there may be certain subgroups in society (e.g., low-income women) who may be at greater risk of obesity because of their lifestyle and circumstances. It is also possible, but not probable in view of the evidence, that there may be a *lag effect*, to the extent that the rise in obesity is the result of societal transformations that have occurred many years ago, but are only now manifesting themselves. At this juncture, our only conclusion must be that we need to look further to uncover a compelling answer to this paradox – which brings us invariably to the eating habits of North Americans.

Fast Food Super-Sized!

Against popular perception, there is both good news and bad news associated with the eating habits of Canadians. According to research by the Agricultural Division of Health Canada, over the last 25 years, the eating habits of Canadians have improved in several key areas. For instance, we eat more vegetables and fruits – the consumption rate in 1997 has increased 27% from the early 1970s (Alain, 1999). In addition, consumption of lower-fat milk has increased; for example, the consumption of 1% fat milk has climbed from 12% of the population in 1990 to 27% in 1997. Also, the eating of red meat has declined slightly. But the good news largely ends here.

Research examining eating habits of Canadians in the late 1990s reveals some disturbing trends. Starkey, Johnson-Down, and Gray-Donald (2001) compared food intake among a random sample of Canadians aged 13 to 65 to the recommended levels found in *Canada's Food Guide to Healthy Eating*. They discovered that only males aged 13 to 34 met the minimum recommended levels of all four of the major food categories (grain products, milk products, meat and alternatives, and vegetables and fruits). Thus, many Canadians are not consuming adequate amounts of food from the major 'healthy food groups' that contain iron, calcium, folates, vitamin C, vitamin A, zinc, and other important vitamins and minerals. Although some of these can be obtained through vitamin supplements, the data suggest that most Canadians are demonstrating unhealthy eating habits. It is striking that these researchers discovered that over 25% of energy burned by both adolescents and adults originates from the 'Other Food Group' (the largest contributor of any food group), which includes soft drinks and fruit drinks, desserts, donuts, candies, ice cream bars, potato chips, oils, spreads, and similar types of foods (Starkey, et al., 2001). Furthermore, the proportion of energy connected to these unhealthy foods would be even larger if French fries were included in this list rather than being categorized with vegetables and fruits, since French fries are high in polysaturated fats and fit better within the unhealthy group.

But one should also ask whether longitudinal studies support these findings. Indeed, research conducted on eating patterns over time confirms the results from cross-sectional studies based on recent eating habits. North Americans have experienced an alarming escalation in the consumption of soft drinks, which contain few nutrients and considerable amounts of sugar. According to Alain (1999), the average number of litres of pop per person in the United States has almost doubled between 1975 and 1997, from about 60 litres to 106 litres per person per year. In his book, *Fast Food Nation*, Schlosser (2002) similarly shows that over the last four decades, the per capita consumption of carbonated soft drinks has quadrupled. There also has been a significant rise in the number of oils and fats consumed in various foods, some of which are high in saturated fat (low-density lipids), and therefore contribute to high overall cholesterol levels. Use of oils in salads has also grown – albeit some contain olive oil and other beneficial high-density fats. However, consumption of oils and trans fatty acids found in deep-fried foods has been on the rise, the oils that typically contain the low-density lipid cholesterol and fatty acids that are associated with heart disease and diabetes. Recent studies also suggest that these deep fried oils may be carcinogenic. A highly publicized Swedish study has shown that the chemical acrylamide significantly increases the risk of cancer in animals. Acrylamide is used in plastics and is produced when certain oils are heated to high temperatures, as they are in the making of French fries, potato chips, and cereals.

There is also evidence that eating outside the home has become more commonplace, and that this type of eating is connected to the quality and quantity of food consumed. Struempler (2002) notes that Americans eat 1 out of every 5 meals outside the home, and, moreover, that 4 out of 10 of these are fast food meals. And it is understood that eating patterns in Canada are beginning to mirror those in the United States, as part of a North American trend. To make matters worse, there has been a move towards super-sized servings in certain restaurants. This has been occurring in virtually all fast food outlets. Today, the average meal in a restaurant is 2 to 3 times the meal size recommended by the United States Department of Agriculture (USDA). But the fast food industry is probably the largest contributor to oversized food portions. According to Kendall (2000), in the 1950s a serving of McDonald's French fries was about 2 ounces, whereas today it is about 5 ounces, and an order of what the company called its Super Sized Fries was 3 times as large. In addition, hamburgers have grown in size from about 1 ounce to between 4 and 10 ounces over that same period, and soft drink sizes have doubled to tripled in volume. Even muffins, bagels, and other grain products have been super-sized, so that even though you may select a healthy food group, the portion size is too large. Furthermore, Schlosser (2002) reports that the size of carbonated soft drinks at fast food restaurants have swelled from eight ounces in the late 1950s to 12 ounces today for a child's drink, and a shocking 32 ounces (p. 241) for a large adult drink. The fact that the fast food industry has begun to permeate public and post-secondary school environments is indicative that simply providing information about what constitutes healthy living is not enough to break the current eating patterns.

The most comprehensive longitudinal analysis of trends in standardized food portion sizes has been recently published in the *Journal of the American Medical Association* (Nielsen and Popkin, 2003). Although comparisons are not made as far back as the 1950s, the data cover the period between the late 1970s and the 1990s and are the most reliable for estimating changing food portion sizes. Using a large representative sample of 63,380 persons aged 2 and over from two U.S. surveys – the Nationwide Food Consumption Survey (1977–78) and the Continuing Survey of Food Intake by Individuals (1989–91, 1994–96, and 1998) – researchers measured average portion sizes for many of the foods considered to be contributing to the obesity rate in North America. These foods were then linked to eating location – home, restaurant, or fast food outlet. The foods in this group include salty snacks, desserts, soft drinks,

French fries, hamburgers, cheeseburgers, pizza, and Mexican food, most of which fall under the 'Other Food Group' category in Canada's food guide.

Nielsen and Popkin (2003) also discovered that the largest portions of food were consumed at fast food establishments, followed by the home, and, finally, at non-fast food restaurants. Moreover, between 1977 and 1996, statistically significant increases were found in total food portion sizes consumed for all food groups listed above, except for pizza. Specifically, over this 20-year period, the average portion size for all eating environments increased 60% for salty snacks, 52% for soft drinks, 27% for Mexican food, 22% for hamburgers, and 16% for French fries. Yet, the bulging portions observed for the period between 1977 and 1996 were even greater for fast food outlets – the average portion size increased 58% for salty snacks, 62% for soft drinks, 37% for Mexican food, 18% for hamburgers, and 57% for French fries. To add fuel to the fire, it is well known in this research literature that self-reports of portion sizes significantly underestimate true levels, and that under-reporting has increased over time.

A major study conducted by Binkley et al. (2000) provides even further elaboration of the associations between where we eat and unhealthy body weight. Using data from the 1994–96 U.S. Continuing Survey of Food Intake by Individuals (CSFII), a nationally representative sample of 16,103 individuals, these researchers specifically investigated the relationship between the source from which food has been obtained and obesity in adults. The researchers used a measure of the proportion of total grams of food purchased at restaurants, and another measure for the proportion of total grams of food purchased at fast food outlets, over the 24 hours preceding the survey. In addition, a number of other known correlates of obesity were incorporated into a multivariate analysis, including age, gender, education, income, ethnicity, unemployment, smoking, exercise, health status, television watching, region, total energy consumption, and whether a person was on a diet or was a vegetarian. It was found that fast food sources predict obesity in both men and women, and that other restaurant sources predict obesity for men only. Thus, at least using cross-sectional data, there is evidence that eating fast food is correlated positively with obesity, even after statistically controlling for an extensive list of potentially confounding variables. Furthermore, eating in restaurants has the same negative effect, but apparently only for men.

A number of other variables examined in this study also presented associations with obesity (Binkley et al., 2000). Of particular interest to this discussion is the influence of exercise, perceived health, smoking status, and television watching on obesity. Noteworthy are the strong findings for vigorous exercise and healthy weight, which is consistent with other literature on predictors of obesity. A weak finding is observed for television watching and being over-weight, which fits with our previous conclusion pertaining to the role of television for obesity.

Thus, super-sizing in the fast food industry both at restaurants and in the home has probably been most responsible for oversized portions. Researchers have identified the relative pricing of larger portions of fast food as one primary reason for this consumption pattern. Yet, individuals ultimately make the decision to overeat; thus, the attributes of consumers and those connected to the supply and marketing of food, as well as those embedded in broader societal change, need to be placed into the causal formula. This point is reflected in the fact that unhealthy portion sizes are also occurring in the food decisions made at home. Moreover, these profound patterns in the quantity and quality of food consumed by individuals and families are consistent with the rise in obesity.

Our analyses of socio-economic status, region, and lifestyle factors among baby boomers also established some additional obesity patterns relevant to this discussion. Although the income differential in obesity is only about 10%, it has been rising at a faster rate in the lower-income group than in the higher-income one. Thus, there is some evidence of a culture of poverty that generates disadvantage, in this case unhealthy body weight and health risk because of the absence of economic resources. In *Fast Food Nation*, Schlosser (2002) con-tends that the fast food industry originally targeted persons of lower socio-economic status, providing them with an affordable restaurant experience. However, more recently, fast food has been marketed to children, adults, and families from all segments of society, which is also apparent in our data. With respect to education, it is interesting that we also found a 20% higher obesity rate among persons not having post-secondary education (compared to their counterparts), but the importance of this factor has been waning over time, rather than rising. The education effect may be declining, in part, because obesity (and probably the eating habits connected to it) is cutting across all major groupings in North America. We also found that obesity exhibits a number of regional variations, where it has been escalating faster in Ontario than in the Prairie provinces over the last two decades but is currently highest in the Maritimes and lowest in Quebec and BC. Regional trends likely reflect key cultural, socio-economic status, and ethnic differentiation across the coun-try. Furthermore, foreign-born persons of boomer age were one-third less likely to be obese than Canadian-born boomers. Overall, while these socio-economic status, regional, and foreign-born status patterns in obesity are salient, what is most striking is that obesity has become an epidemic – perme-ating all sectors of society. In other words, we are fast becoming an oversized nation, and one that appears to be slipping from the ranks of the healthy nations of the world.

Explaining Food Consumption Patterns

So, why do progressively more individuals in society eat in ways that are unhealthy? Like all health behaviours, eating is complex and multifarious. However, we can point to a few primary reasons based on a review of the research. There is agreement in the literature that both work stressors and life stressors are proliferating. We work longer and at a faster pace than ever before in an increasingly global economic marketplace that is highly competitive. Often multiple family members work to maintain or improve family income levels and standard of living. This is evidenced by the fact that the labour force participation of women has risen dramatically, from about 37% in 1970 to 57% in 1997 (Federal, Provincial and Territorial Advisory Committee on Population Health, 1999). Additionally, it has been estimated that between 1991 and 1995, there was a significant increase in rates of work-related stress reported by workers, especially women, and particularly those who are single parents. When people are busy and stressed, they likely eat fast foods more often, both in and out of the home. It is easier to pick up a bucket of chicken and a box of French fries or order a pizza than to shop for the ingredients and cook a dinner covering all of the major food groups, especially when you are a working single mother or father, or a working couple. Also, many fast foods taste better than more healthy ones. However, foods that can be cooked and consumed quickly are typically high in polysaturated fats and often are missing important nutrients. It is revealing that about 13% of Canadians stated in a recent survey that they did not have time to prepare a healthy meal, while 74% stated that they eat in a hurry, and 39% of employed people stated that they consume meals in a vehicle because of busy work schedules (Federal, Provincial, and Territorial Advisory Committee on Population Health, 1999).

Another pertinent question is why are people not getting the message? Although health promotion information available through media channels has proliferated recently, especially with Internet access, some people appear to be confused by conflicting health messages. This is probably most apparent for nutritional and diet recommendations. The moment a study supports an association between a particular food and an illness, it finds its way onto the front page of a newspaper or magazine. This is problematic, of course, because one study is not adequate scientific proof and replication of any finding is a fundamental and agreed upon requirement. Also, coverage of medical findings in the media rarely offer evaluations of methodology or place findings in the context of the knowledge base in the specific field. Research into media messaging has long shown that multiple complex messages confuse individuals. For instance, over recent years the media have reported that eggs are bad for one's health because of their cholesterol content, and have then followed with the message that eggs are good because they are a source of vitamin E and omega-3 fatty acids. We also have been exposed to a variety of communications channels that tell us that some low-fat versions of foods, such as potato chips, may be carcinogenic. Adding to this information pot, we have been alerted to research suggesting that people who are obese are happier, not to mention that chocolate makes us feel better. Although Health Canada provides scientifically supported nutritional guidelines and information about diets, this health knowledge is diluted by the popular press and individuals' natural reluctance to invest the time and energy necessary to initiate and sustain significant changes to unhealthy lifestyles, if they are prone to them. Therefore, while facilitation of awareness, knowledge, and attitudes is important, these must be combined with the motivation, skills, time, and capacity needed to change lifestyle behaviours.

Furthermore, there are literally thousands of diets, each with its own theory and approach to weight reduction. For example, recent attention has been given to high-protein, low-carbohydrate diets, such as the Atkins and the South Beach Diets, ones that stand out as contradictory to popular notions of healthy eating habits. We typically hear that we should be eating at least 5 to 6 portions of fruit, vegetables, and whole grains per day, rather than raising consumption of foods high in protein, particularly meats. Although there is mounting evidence that a high-protein diet is very effective in weight reduction, there is a paucity of long-term studies on the potential deleterious consequences of such a diet. Preliminary findings point to possible negative consequences for the liver and kidneys if the high-protein phase of this diet is followed for an extended period of time. Moreover, the long-term success rates for many diets are typically not studied, or not made known to the public.

Yet, there is ample evidence that diets high in fresh fruit and vegetables – those that contain fewer processed foods and smaller amounts of foods from the 'Other Food Group' as noted in Canada's food guide, and which entail balance in the other food groups – will provide sufficient healthy nutrients as well as body weight maintenance (Binkley et al., 2000; Jeffery and French, 1998). Such diets will also reduce serum lipids that contribute to high cholesterol (Jenkins et al., 1997). Moreover, fats with high-density lipids – those in what is known as the Mediterranean diet, which uses olive oil, and, typically, fish containing omega-3 fatty acids – have beneficial effects on our cardiovascular system. For instance, Hu et al. (2000) have established in a large-sample longitudinal study that a 'prudent diet' significantly decreases the incidence of non-fatal myocardial infarction and fatal coronary heart disease. This diet includes higher intake of vegetables, fruit, legumes, whole grains, fish and poultry, and is similar to the Mediterranean Diet. The less healthy 'Western diet' entails greater amounts of red meat, processed meat, refined grains, sweets and desserts, French fries, and high-fat dairy products. Another large-sample study of Greek subjects compared their Mediterranean diet to a Western one (Hu, 2003), finding that a traditional Greek diet increased longevity by 25%. The Mediterranean diet consists of the same foods as the 'prudent diet,' but it also emphasizes consumption of olives and olive oil, nuts, and moderate red wine with most meals, and only small amounts of red meats.

Unfortunately, healthy foods and diets are not always the most appealing. Conversely, fast foods often taste good and are readily available. Moreover, healthy food-consumption messages targeting the public must battle advertising messages that implore them to consume unhealthy quantities or types of food. The presentation of products, especially fast food, has become a multi-million-dollar industry that has developed highly effective methods to make these foods irresistible (Schlosser, 2002). In a free market system in which profit and sustainability of industry are the primary goals, lifestyle messages must compete on an uneven playing field. In this sense, the problem is systemic, fraught with social, political, and economic barriers and pitfalls.

Physical Activity: We Still Have a Long Way to Go

Even though the evidence suggests that Canadians, including baby boomers, enjoy more healthy levels of exercise and physical activity than two decades ago by meeting minimum recommended guidelines, there is considerable room for improvement. Developing and sustaining an active lifestyle shares many of the same facets as eating habits – awareness, knowledge, attitudes, intentions, motivation, skills, time, and capacity to change. It should be noted that 57% of the population aged 12 and over reported physical activity levels deemed to be in the inactive category (less than 1.5 kilocalories used per kilogram of body weight per day), according to the 1996/97 National Population Health Survey. Furthermore, only 7% of the population aged 15 and over walk to work and only 1% ride a bicycle (Federal, Provincial and Territorial Advisory Committee on Population Health, 1999).

As shown in this book, unhealthy exercise levels affect persons of all ages and sexes. Based on the recent 2000/01 Canadian Community Health Survey, once people reach their mid-20s, the rate of unhealthy exercise (defined in this book as not meeting conservative minimum guidelines) hovers around the

40% mark for most age groups. Although this is an improvement over the 1978/79 rate of 60%, we still have a long way to go to reach the exercise levels observed in some European countries. Moreover, there remain a number of target groups whose activity levels stand out. For instance, it appears that young women are particularly prone to an inactive lifestyle. Additionally, a comparison of baby boomers today with persons their age two decades ago demonstrated that persons of lower education (high school or less) exhibited a 21% higher rate of unhealthy exercise than those with post-secondary education. A similar pattern in unhealthy exercise was uncovered for low-income persons. Also, a clear east-west gradient was found, whereby rates of unhealthy exercise declined moving from the Maritimes to British Columbia. It was also observed that Canadian-born boomers reported 10% lower rates of unhealthy exercise compared to foreign-born individuals.

Clearly, the most salient trend is the fact that the proportion of the population below these minimum recommended levels of exercise, in any of these subgroups, is simply too high. However, an emphasis on simply improving exercise levels in society in order to solve the obesity epidemic is not supported by research. Cross-sectional and panel analyses indicate that while exercise is a predictor of obesity, the relationship is not as strong as what one might expect, and, furthermore, that it is overshadowed by a number of other lifestyle factors not the least of which entails eating habits (Binkley et al., 2000). In fact, examination of the association between obesity and exercise among boomers, based on the 2001 CCHS, shows that 19.3% of obese (BMI 30+) baby boomers were exercising at the unhealthy level, whereas 14.8% exercised above that level. This is only a difference of 4.5 percentage points, and a 30% higher rate of obesity among the unhealthy exercise group. In other words, the likelihood of being obese is probably affected by exercise level, but its influence is modest. Taken together, it is clear that we must focus on more than a singular lifestyle behaviour to address this public health problem. When activity patterns are combined with progressively unhealthy eating habits and body weights, it becomes obvious that we have a long way to go for the average Canadian to be considered as having a healthy lifestyle, or for us to boast that we are a healthy nation.

Reflections on the Exercise-Obesity Paradox

One of the unanticipated costs of a high-paced life indeed may be the development of poor eating habits. We simply eat more food than needed, and we consume too many foods that are unhealthy and not easily burned through exercise. These patterns have both short- and long-term detrimental effects on our health. We also are not first internalizing and then acting on the healthy eating and activity messages. This is a problem that will not be corrected by modest advances in physical activity levels alone, especially when the absolute exercise level needed in Canada is not being met. Thus, alterations in both food consumption and exercise patterns are required to reverse the obesity phenomenon.

Few government policies prioritize the importance of nutrition, diet, and exercise in a manner that is powerful and effective. Certainly, Health Canada and many other groups publish recommended levels and guidelines; however, these are not having a significant impact on behaviour as yet, and they certainly are not counteracting the negative influential elements in society. A more aggressive approach to encourage healthy diets and activity levels is desperately needed. In tandem with strong, effective media campaigns, there needs to be specific healthy public policies dealing with the environment to foster more active lifestyles. This might include green spaces and environments that are conducive to physical activity, such as walking and using bicycle paths in urban areas. These and other health policy changes are discussed further in Chapter 12.

The Lifestyle-Health Status Paradox

Due to the efforts of the 'new public health,' there is the perception that we are making marked improvements in reducing chronic illnesses, especially cardiovascular disease. If healthy lifestyles are a problem for North Americans, then why are rates of cardiovascular disease dropping and why are some other chronic diseases waning as well? As reported in this volume, persons aged 45 to 64 have exhibited substantial reductions in the prevalence rates for arthritis/rheumatism, hypertension, cardiovascular disease, and bronchitis/emphysema between the late 1970s and the late 1990s (Statistics Canada, 1999b). Countering these trends, however, are striking increases that have occurred in prevalence rates for diabetes, asthma, and migraine headaches, as well as for the total number of chronic conditions. Among the elderly, for whom chronic illness has become prevalent, we have witnessed no improvements for any of the major chronic illnesses for the 20-year period between 1978/79 and, 1998/99, and, moreover, rates of diabetes, dementia, certain cancers, and asthma have actually risen. Therefore, the isolated reductions in some chronic illnesses among midlife persons are offset in part by upswings in the prevalence rates of others. There is some evidence in the literature that there is a compression of morbidity (Fries, 1983; Manuel and Schultz, 2001; Robine et al., 1998), suggesting that the overall health gains over chronic-illness prevalence among the baby boomers will likely continue into their elder years. However, the most interesting story told by our data is that the constellation of chronic conditions faced by different cohorts of individuals as they age is probably going to be more complex and unpredictable, and therefore more important to the health of these individuals than the relatively modest gains in healthy life expectancy. In other words, while people likely will be free of disability for longer periods of their lives due to the continuation of compression of morbidity, there is considerable fluctuation in the physical and cognitive chronic conditions they will invariably experience as they age.

While it is understood that lifestyle behaviours are only one factor in the causal chain of influence for chronic illnesses, they nevertheless have profound implications for these observed patterns. Declining rates of smoking, unhealthy levels of exercise, and heavy drinking appear to correlate with drops in cardiovascular disease prevalence. Furthermore, the inflation of diabetes rates can be connected to the rise in obesity, and in turn may have a negative influence on cardiovascular disease, since diabetes is a major risk factor (CACR, 1999). It is not surprising that obesity is considered to be the new tobacco. Additionally, asthma rates have been linked to deteriorating air quality, while migraine rates may be connected to the compounding life stresses reported by individuals during the last two decades. In this sense, population and cohort-specific shifts in healthy lifestyles are actually consistent with many of the reported trends in specific chronic illnesses.

This apparent paradox between lifestyle change and health status change also requires consideration of other factors that may influence reported prevalence rates of chronic illness. Barer et al. (1995) and Evans et al. (2001) demonstrate that there has been an intensification of health services over two decades, especially among older adults, including significant elevation in the cost of pharmaceuticals, doctor-patient ratios, and hospital services. On the one hand, the lowering of the rate of certain chronic conditions such as hypertension, certain cancers, and arthritis may be due to early detection and the use of pharmacological treatments and other forms of intervention – there can be little argument that we are getting better at preventing, detecting, and treating many chronic illnesses at their onset, which may reduce their long-term prevalence in society separately from lifestyle factors. On the other hand, more sensitive screening methods and technology may inflate the prevalence of certain diseases. For example, evidence-based guidelines for cardiovascular disease and diabetes screening have been broadened, resulting in fewer missed positive diagnoses, but perhaps more false ones as well.

There is some evidence that the public may have become complacent about their health, relying more on the health care system to fix problems when they arise rather than making the necessary changes to health behaviours and sustaining them in order to prevent illness in the first place. One of the recent pharmacological developments is what has been called the Polypill, a new multi-formula medication made up of a cocktail of six compounds: Aspirin, a cholesterol drug, three blood pressure-lowering medications at half the usual dose, and folic acid (Kirkey, 2003). The developers of Polypill intend to prescribe it to anyone aged 55 and over, to significantly reduce risk factors associated with cardiovascular disease. Another family of pharmaceuticals (e.g., Xenical) is being developed to reduce obesity in children and adults in lieu of diet and exercise change. Thus, the proliferation of 'preventive' pharmacological treatments may unintentionally and adversely affect an individual's motivation to maintain a healthy lifestyle. The choice of a pill over making significant alterations to lifestyle behaviours may be too easy for some individuals. This is particularly problematic in a society that has become over-medicalized in a number of ways (Rachlis and Kushner, 1994).

Attempts to make important lifestyle changes may often come too late or are attempted too quickly, with negative consequences. Dr Nicolas DiNubile of the American Academy of Orthopedic Surgeons has coined the term *boomeritis* – the tendency for baby boomers to attempt to remain active but to overuse their bodies in doing so, resulting in musculoskeletal injury (Lee, 2002). This is portrayed as a problem related to the baby boomers' attempts to stay young in the face of aging processes, and trying to do this beyond their physical ability. One major consequence in the United States has been an increase in emergency room visits and MRIs related to this kind of injury among baby boomers. DiNubile further argues that boomeritis can be mitigated by more careful activity regimens, including proper warm-ups, rest, and exercise progression, but that too often boomers are impatient or do not have the time to do the routines required to maintain active lifestyles. This observation points to an underlying problem – the fact that some baby boomers' expectations about health deal more with looking good than with being healthy, which may not necessarily be synonymous.

Food manufacturers have also facilitated a continuation of unhealthy eating habits. Rather than cutting out or significantly reducing consumption of various foods, such as snack foods, with high levels of saturated fats (e.g., potato chips) or other proven unhealthy contents, the availability of low-fat or even 'low-carb' versions allows individuals to continue their eating patterns largely intact. Instead of solving the problem, the low-fat movement is affording the consumer an easy rationalization for unhealthy eating habits, sometimes with unintended negative consequences. The idea that having a balance of foods that meets recommended nutrition levels set out in Canada's food guide has been lost somewhere between the battle among corporations to retain or inflate their portion of global market share, and families' and individuals' adaptation to an increasingly demanding and fast-paced work and leisure life. Clearly, it is going to take more than an array of websites offering health information to motivate individuals, families, and communities to make significant changes to their lifestyle-health behaviours.

12

Health Policy Relevance, Future Scenarios, and Conclusions

The Research–Health Policy Interface

There is a growing awareness that research plays a pivotal role in the construction and revision of health policies. Earlier chapters have featured a number of studies that investigate aspects of healthy lifestyles by means of comparative analyses across two points in time. While findings from those studies are insightful, using any two surveys by themselves – such as only the 1978/79 CHS and 1998/99 NPHS – does not uncover the level of specificity and knowledge required to identify important patterns that may lie ahead. Indeed, using only two points with cross-sectional trend data may mask important shifts in behaviours and outcomes occurring between those dates, and does not afford the opportunity to engage more sophisticated age-period-cohort analysis. The development of detailed health profiles of baby boom cohorts, and our analysis of the three health domains based on several sequential cross-sectional surveys spanning almost two and a half decades (1978/79 – 2000/01), provides a higher level of information for health planning and programming both for today and for the future. Yet, although it sheds new light on the problem, even this level of analysis constitutes only a starting point, and begs further research as a means to support the development of social policy and health promotion programmatic efforts.

The design of policies will have to respond not only to what we know about today's population, but also to the past experiences built into successive cohorts moving through their life cycles, each affected differently by historical events and social change. The Social Change Model provides a dynamic framework for connecting population changes and societal changes, and their manifestation within individual behaviours. Given that the baby boomers are a primary driving force for consumer behaviour for the next several decades

(Foot, 1996; Morgan 1998a,b), it is important to analyse the different cohorts that constitute the baby boom generation. In this book, this includes distinguishing persons within that generation, for example, investigating younger and older boomers as well as gender, socio-economic, regional, and foreign-born status variations. Even though the baby boomers have comprised the focus of this study, the full age spectrum has also been examined where possible. This is imperative, not only to compare and anchor the baby boomer cohorts but also to elucidate nuances occurring among other age-sex groups. Moreover, analyses of all cohorts comprising our age pyramid are necessary to better understand population health. The evolution of these patterns across age, period, and cohort demands consideration of the potentially differential effects of influential historical events and cultural change in Canadian society.

As a starting point, the identification of pervasive age, period, and cohort patterns of lifestyle and socio-demographic determinants of health, indicators of health status, and health utilization alerts policy-makers, researchers, and health organizations to emerging health trends on the horizon. For instance, this research suggests that, while obesity has risen dramatically over the last 15 years for virtually all age groups and cohorts, there are some distinguishable trends. It has doubled for men aged 20 to 64, but has nearly tripled for women in that age group. The rate of obesity also has proliferated faster among younger boomers than among older ones. Additionally, wealthier baby boomers appear to be gaining ground on their counterparts with respect to unhealthy body weight, suggesting a weakening of the income effect and a proliferation of obesity throughout all segments of society. Furthermore, the inflation of obesity rates in these groups has occurred while exercise rates actually have moved in the opposite direction – what we have called the exercise-obesity paradox. We have weighed the value of a number of explanations for this paradox, such as alterations in leisure time and work-related physical activity, television watching, and computer use. Our investigation has led us invariably to changes in food consumption habits, which have devolved significantly beyond what our activity levels have been able to counter.

We recognize that all lifestyle behaviours under examination have multiple determinants, and are interrelated as well. These causal factors include, among other things, the fact that individuals are reflecting fundamental social and cultural transformations. For instance, a faster pace of life; the availability, mass appeal, and affordability of fast foods compared to more healthy ones; the economy of super-sized portion sizes; confusion about what constitutes healthy eating; and the absence of an effective health policy and effective health programs comprise only part of the puzzle. The health consequences of these lifestyle and health trends are enormous, and require massive efforts for their reversal.

Coupled with detailed health profiling, the analyses presented in the previous chapters helped as well to uncover complexity within relationships among variables connected to the different health domains under examination, such as the effect of changing lifestyles, chronic illness, and health care utilization. Significant declines in the prevalence of smoking and heavy drinking, coupled with a drop in unhealthy exercise rates, have led in all likelihood to a decrease in cardiovascular disease and certain cancers. However, the dramatic escalation in obesity probably has contributed to the upturn in diabetes, and likely cancelled some of the benefits gained from improvements in other healthy lifestyles, such as regular and sufficient physical activity. The continuation of a highly medicalized population is perhaps less surprising in the face of these trends, but carries with it certain consequences for society, such as over-reliance on pharmaceuticals to reduce risk factors for, and management of, illness that may be controlled through alterations in lifestyle. However, the trend towards what essentially is medicalization of unhealthy lifestyles is not surprising, given that the pharmaceutical industry has become one of the fastest growing multinationals in the global market.

Additionally, the results of this research elucidate often hidden, unanticipated health patterns that may have significant consequences for our health system. This information is vital given that the front end of the baby boom will move into its senior years in 2011. The contention that the baby boomers have a 'poor report card' and therefore will become a burden to society once they age has not been supported. Nor is the view that baby boomers are healthier and wealthier, thus substantially reducing any future potential deleterious effect on our health care system. Indeed the story is much more colourful. First, baby boomers are not a homogeneous group, but rather demonstrate considerable variation in health dynamics across cohort, gender, and a number of other socio-demographic factors. Second, although we are observing broadening prevalence of chronic illnesses over time, including a substantial rise in diabetes, it is just as important to consider how the organization, growth, and development of the health care system influences health. Predicting utilization patterns of the baby boomers during their golden years may have as much to do with their attitudes and with health care reform as it does with analysing health and illness profiles. Based on some of the data presented, one could surmise that baby boomers will know and expect more out of the health care system than the previous generation, regardless of whether these expectations can be met. Health care reform will need to address efficiency and effectiveness in the health care system in order to accommodate these demands. This includes, among other things, support of health promotion efforts from within the health care system, such as greater emphasis on lifestyle change by the primary care system.

Overall, identification of the ebbs and flows of mutable lifestyle factors, such as physical activity, smoking, drinking, and eating habits, tells us in no uncertain terms that we are failing in our efforts to make Canada a country in which healthy lifestyles are the norm. It is imperative that we, as a nation, carefully scrutinize these emerging trends and take steps to support a healthier population as we become substantially older as a society. So, what have we been doing and what is in store?

Assessing National Programs Targeting Lifestyles

There is at least indirect evidence that national programs targeting lifestyle behaviours can be effective. The ParticipAction program, a non-profit organization started in 1971 by Pierre Trudeau, quickly became a household name. The thrust of the program was a strong media campaign that attempted to embarrass Canadians at all ages for their low-exercise rates, compared to several European countries, and to challenge them to improve their activity levels. It also generated over $40 million in private-sector support to fund various ParticipAction programs. In 1995, 89% of Canadians were aware of the agency and 65% stated that it had influenced their exercise behaviour. However, it is surprising that between 1971 and 2000, the program was run on a total of only $21 million, or less than $1 million a year (Foss, 2000). Moreover, since the mid-1990s, Health Canada has decided to cut the ParticipAction budget from $1 million to only $200,000 in the fiscal year 1999/2000. In November 2001, ParticipAction, an independent, not-for-profit organization, announced it would cease operations on 31 December 2001. Since that time, ParticipAction has remained incorporated, with only a volunteer board of directors, but it is possible that it could be resurrected some time in the future.

The SummerActive Program is a national, community-based, communications campaign designed to raise awareness about the importance of physical fitness, healthy eating, and a tobacco-free lifestyle. Developed by Allan Rock when he was the minister of Health in 2002, the program may have been intended to be a partial replacement for ParticipAction. The program runs between May and June, and was designed to link up with the first WHO Annual Move for Health Day, 10 May 2003. However, the SummerActive Program in its current form likely will not reach enough individuals in an effective manner to have a significant population health effect.

Health Canada (1998b), in association with the Canadian Society for Exercise Physiology, released and distributed the *Canadian Physical Activity Guide to Healthy Active Living*, followed by its sister document aimed at older adults, entitled, *Handbook for Canada's Physical Activity Guide to Healthy Active Living for Older Adults* (Health Canada, 1998c). These documents are the first of their kind in Canada to provide specific, evidence-based recommendations pertaining to the maintenance of an active lifestyle (Spence et al., 2001). The ideal dose of activity recommended is equivalent to 60 minutes daily of any intensity of activity, 30 minutes of moderate-intense activity 4 days a week, or 20 minutes of vigorous-intensity activity 4 days a week (Canadian Fitness and Lifestyle Research Institute, 1998). As yet, the impact of these documents on population health has not been fully appraised.

Concurrently, the federal and provincial governments appear to be poised to shift their focus to multiple healthy lifestyle factors, in particular in the areas of obesity and physical activity. In 2002, the federal, provincial and territorial health ministers announced they were developing what has been called the Integrated Pan-Canadian Healthy Living Strategy, a program that emphasizes lifestyle behaviours. The government of Canada convened its first national summit, called the Healthy Living Symposium, in Toronto on 16–17 June, 2003. The summit was intended to act as part of the consultation process in order to feed into the development of the action plan. It is also closely tied to a new report entitled Improving the Health of Canadians, issued by the Canadian Population Health Initiative of the Canadian Institute for Health Information (CIHI, 2004). To date, the Integrated Pan-Canadian Healthy Living Strategy is composed of invited reports from selected organizations and research communities in support of its development. As well, a discussion document has been written which states that the ministers of health have agreed that the Phase 1 strategy of the action plan will focus on healthy eating and physical activity and their relationship to healthy weights (Federal, Provincial and Territorial Ministers of Health, 2003). It states that

The Integrated Pan-Canadian Healthy Living Strategy is an intersectoral initiative designed to improve health outcomes and reduce disparities in health status in Canada. It is based on a conceptual framework for sustained action ... The strategy is founded on a population health approach and collaborative efforts to promote health and prevent disease and injury. Phase 1 of the strategy focuses on physical activity, health eating and their relationship to healthy weights. Future phases may focus on other priority issues and may include mental health, injury prevention or other important areas of emphasis. (p. 5)

This strategy stems from Canada's central involvement in and endorsement, in May 2000, of the World Health Organization's Global Strategy for the Prevention and Control of Non-communicable Diseases. The WHO strategy targets tobacco, unhealthy diet, and physical inactivity (WHO, 2000). It is interesting that the Canadian strategy has been to choose to address only the latter two factors, at least in Phase 1. Furthermore, the goals of this strategy are similar to those of the famous Ottawa Charter – to reduce health disparities and improve overall health outcomes – as well as to those of the Population Health Model discussed in Chapter 2. However, the uniqueness of the current strategy is the connection between healthy eating and physical activity as common risk factors affecting chronic disease, and the commitment to target these lifestyle factors simultaneously and systematically. This is a marked departure from the typically fragmented programs in the past that have tended to respond to one lifestyle factor at a time, such as the Tobacco Reduction Strategy, or to one particular disease, such as the Heart Health Initiative. The question is whether and to what extent there will be investment of time, effort, and new resources into the realization of the goals articulated within these strategies? Previously lofty goals, such as the 1986 Ottawa Charter's aim to achieve health for all Canadians by the year 2000, have fallen well short according to evidence in the research literature.

The findings stemming from this book are supportive of an integrative approach to healthy living. But there is no doubt that the absence of tobacco from the target list of the Integrated Pan-Canadian Healthy Living Strategy is disturbing, especially given that about one in five Canadians and one in four baby boomers continue to smoke regularly, and that tobacco products constitute a major risk factor for a number of diseases. Moreover, there appears to be mounting attention directed at children and youth, both in terms of the supporting trends and the current Healthy Living Strategy. Although an inclusive life stage approach is adopted in the action plan that lists pre- and post-natal children, youth, midlife adults, and older adults, Phase 1 of the strategy selects only children and youth, as well as Aboriginal peoples, for special emphasis. It is to this issue that we now turn.

Health Promotion and Aging: It's Never Too Late

One of the questions that arises for policy and program development is, Who should be targeted? The notion that healthy lifestyles are the product of life chances and choices culminating over a person's life have been interpreted in different ways. For some, there appears to be an assumption that the greatest 'value added' in our health promoting efforts will be realized among persons who are younger, given that benefits of health promotion action will be experienced for a longer period than for older persons. However, an overemphasis on health behaviours earlier in life can actually devalue and deter health policies and action for lifestyle maintenance and modification among persons in midlife and those reaching advanced ages. The research in this book demonstrates definitively that both improvements and declines in lifestyle behaviours have occurred among persons of all ages, and therefore lifestyle behaviours are mutable across the age spectrum. Yet, there continues to be a focus on children and youth in many of our health promotion efforts. Unquestionably, investments into population health at younger ages will have longer benefits, although it may be true as well that omitting other age groups, especially the elderly, decreases the efficacy of such action. In other words, multifaceted health promotion approaches that can be tailored to, or cut across, particular ages, as well as across gender, socio-economic status, ethnocultural groups, and so on, will likely prove the most effective in terms of overall population health (Wister, 2003).

Indeed, Lalive d'Epinay and Bickel's study (2003) supports a causal link between sport/exercise trajectories measured between midlife (close to age 50) and 'young-old' (aged 65 to 74) and psychological well-being outcomes at these later ages. Specifically, they find that new exercisers in old age rate their health at levels close to those of the long-term exercisers. This result gives credence to the idea that individuals can make up for lost ground, at least with respect to the social-psychological benefits of exercise and perhaps physical ones as well (Wister, 2003). Thus, it is never too late when it comes to improving healthy lifestyles.

So, what is it that is keeping us from developing and sustaining active, healthy lifestyles across the life cycle? There is an enormous literature that addresses the causal mechanisms underlying physical activity patterns (see, for example, Sherwood and Jeffery, 2000). It is understood that physical activity is a complex, dynamic process that is influenced by a large constellation of individual, social, and environmental characteristics. Drawing on various theoretical developments, such as the Developmental Theory, the Health Belief Model, the Theory of Planned Behaviour, the Social Learning Theory, the Transtheoretical Model, the Social Ecological Model, and various social resource perspectives, researchers have identified a list of barriers and facilitators to physical activity processes. These have occurred at the societal level (e.g., economic, normative, and cultural factors), community level (e.g., marginalization processes, availability of sports facilities, parks, walkways, and green spaces), and at individual and family levels (e.g., socio-demographic and SES factors, motivation, intention, stage of change, health knowledge, and beliefs). What can be gleaned from this literature is that a multi-pronged approach to active living that recognizes the heterogeneity of people of all ages is probably going to produce the greatest population health gains.

Such an approach necessitates expansion of targeted health promotion pro-grams that meet the needs, resources, and readiness to change of individuals at various points in the life course, individuals with different attitude and belief systems (e.g., related to culture, gender, and SES), individuals with different health conditions and those living in different places and under different circumstances. The development of an active lifestyle should start early, at which point people are probably the most malleable. Obviously school-, peer-, and family-based programs are paramount in order to promote an early understanding of what constitutes a healthy lifestyle, healthy patterns of eating and physical activity, and ways to maintain them. Children constitute a major focus of health promotion around the time their peer groups become more salient in their lives. The understanding of peer group dynamics and how to utilize these in a positive way could be fruitful for a number of lifestyle behaviours besides tobacco prevention or cessation strategies, which appear to have decreased teenage smoking recently. Concentrating on raising the physi-cal activity component of school curricula coupled with better food options in the school environment may have long-term lifestyle benefits. Indeed, the rapid rise in obesity and the upturn in doctor visits and pharmaceutical use among teenagers is suggestive of unsuccessful health promotion efforts, or a recession of programs that concentrate on these groups.

The period of life in which individuals are young adults (ages 19–35) is also important because many patterns of behaviour are defined more permanently during this period. Higher education is becoming the norm for many young adults; however, physical education is not mandatory in colleges and universi-ties. Rather, the individual is expected to take responsibility for his or her own lifestyle choices. Additionally, this is a time when people seek to establish their independence and begin to form and build families, as well as pursue their work lives. These competing spheres reflect a stage that tends to involve significant fluctuations in life circumstances, increasing financial and social pressures, and greater expectations, which may impede the development or maintenance of healthy lifestyles. Although persons in their 20s tend to enjoy the highest rates of physical activity, by the time they move into their 30s, the maintenance of healthy lifestyles appears to become more problematic, as evidenced in the changing prevalence rates. Programs that attempt to sustain levels of activity and reduce smoking and heavy drinking, and those that support healthy eating during this period in the life course, need to recognize these challenges. Making healthy lifestyles appear fun, attractive, and normal may raise motivation in young adults.

Midlife persons have comprised a major focus of this book because of questions such as, Are the baby boomers healthier than previous generations? While we have provided a partial answer to this particular question, many stones remain unturned. The midlife stage is crucial because it is the period when work and family become major forces. It is also a time when people pass through their physiological peak. All too often, individuals accept the notion that it is normative to become overweight and to decrease activity levels after age 40 or so. Thus, it is important not only to provide people with the knowledge and resources to continue healthy lifestyles as they age, but also to target high-risk groups (e.g., those with a constellation of risk factors for cardiovascular disease, diabetes, or cancer) in health promotion efforts. Altering the social norms surrounding healthy and unhealthy lifestyles is also a cornerstone for any health promotion approach that aims to permeate our heterogeneous, multicultural society.

Turning to older adults, structured exercise programs may benefit by anticipating a certain degree of dropout, and by improving methods of recruiting and maintaining participants who are experiencing aging-related changes or symptoms of illness (Prohaska, 1998). Activity programs need to be enjoyable, appear attractive to individuals with different tastes and preferences, and amalgamate social components in order to reinforce commitment and continued involvement. Health professionals also need to be more intensely involved in supporting the adoption and/or continuation of healthy lifestyles of all kinds, given their influential position in the health care system. Moreover, they should be prepared to assist individuals in understanding best-practice guidelines pertaining to exercise and diet, as well as the intricacies of medication interactions, especially among older adults managing a chronic illness or a constellation of illnesses, which is not uncommon.

At a broader level, there is little doubt that attitudes in society must change. With respect to physical activity, efforts to improve levels significantly among persons of all ages through national campaigns need to recognize the necessity of making exercise part of a lifestyle that can be supported through young adulthood and midlife and into older adulthood. At a health policy level, there needs to be greater commitment by governments to make an active society a priority. The construction and organization of safe bikeways and walkways, green spaces, and parks are examples of ways that the built environment can be manipulated in a way to facilitate active lifestyles – for instance, in the Netherlands bicycles are a frequent mode of transportation for persons of all ages. But this requires investment of financial resources, and not just from the public sphere. What we have learned from smoking campaigns is that the industries that are responsible, even in part, for health problems must be held accountable. It may be possible, therefore, to translate this approach to the fast food industry. In fact, McDonald's has incorporated more healthy food choices into its menu, and has announced that it will discontinue the super-sizing of fast food meals. (Whether this is because of social pressures or a response to a dwindling share of the fast food market is currently difficult to ascertain.) Moreover, understanding the linkages among lifestyle behaviours such as diet, smoking, and exercise may help in the design of programs that prioritize multiple lifestyle factors in an effective manner. In sum, it is imperative that we propagate a positive message that teaches individuals to begin as early as possible, but that it is never too late to adopt or kick-start a healthy lifestyle. It is important as well to understand the potential role, not only of government but also of the private sector, in population and public health efforts.

So What Is a Healthy Lifestyle?

One of the starting points in this book was a definition of a healthy lifestyle, whereby we drew from the more widely known *lifestyle approach* found in the health literature to construct a working definition. It was stated earlier that the ways in which people initiate and maintain healthy lifestyles is a lifelong process that is shaped by complex and dynamic systems interacting among physiological, psychological, and social domains. A healthy lifestyle, and the specific health behaviours that comprise it – a sufficient physical activity level, healthy eating habits, no smoking, and reasonable alcohol consumption – are influenced by a person's social status, social expectations, and health beliefs (Wister, 1996). Thus, we cannot separate healthy lifestyles from the social context in which they are manifested. A healthy lifestyle also entails commitment to either maintaining or adopting behavioural patterns that are shown to have a positive influence on health status. These must be routinized into our daily lives in such a way as to make them easy to replicate over significant periods of time, allowing their health benefits to be realized. Furthermore, it needs to be understood that a healthy lifestyle is not the result of a singular behaviour, but is rather the interactions of many interwoven behavioural patterns. For example, an individual who exercises at a level that produces its full effect and eats healthy foods, but who smokes, is cancelling or reversing the beneficial outcomes and thus is not following a healthy lifestyle.

Health promotion policies and programmatic efforts need to be formulated, organized, and implemented in a way that recognizes the multiplicity and interconnectedness of lifestyle behaviours and understands their aetiology and mutability. While this appears straightforward on the surface, adding this level of complexity to healthy public policy and program development requires a new perspective – one that views healthy lifestyles as behaviours that transcend individual choice and responsibility. That is not to say that individual responsibility should not be a key component in health promotion campaigns, but that it must not be the only one. The situational and social context of individuals, families, or communities being targeted needs to be considered carefully; for example, the presence or absence of various resources, or the cultural facets of a particular group.

In reviewing literature on this topic, one of the most simple but powerful messages is that infusing balance in one's lifestyle is pivotal to good health; that balancing stress and relaxation, activity, diet and eating habits, body and mind, individual responsibility, and awareness of barriers to changing health behaviours are all part of a healthy lifestyle. Such an approach is not automatic; it is learned and relearned through various interpersonal and institutional channels as we age. It is also something that may not come easily to individuals who are facing stressful conditions in life, with few social or financial resources to facilitate change, or few opportunities for introspection. There is no singular formula that will be effective for everyone, but there are lifestyle axioms that are identifiable and reachable for large segments of society, including the marginalized and disadvantaged. We know that strength training combined with aerobic exercise has enormous health benefits, and even walking can improve cardiovascular health significantly (Manson et al., 2002). We know that the quality and quantity of foods influence our health. And we know that smoking and heavy drinking are deleterious. Achieving incremental improvement in healthy lifestyles for enough people may prove to be one simple and effective strategy for population health. For instance, we have witnessed the implementation of walking programs at community and national levels in North America, as well as the proliferation of pedometer devices and programs targeting individuals, such as the 1,000-steps-a-day walking program (Wister, 1999). Why can't walking become a fad?

There is no doubt that we as a society have not realized the full power inherent in propagating a healthy lifestyle norm that truly can be part of the culture of a country. This is especially true in Canada, a country that is still developing its unique national identity, and one that could benefit from the incorporation of healthy lifestyles as a core principle. Uncovering these fundamental aspects of healthy lifestyles is dependent on significant investment in research, policy, and action.

Limitations, Research Gaps, and Challenges

The research presented in this book provides a stepping stone for future work in this area. There are, however, several limitations that temper the conclusions of this research. First, the measures used for the age-period-cohort analyses are only crude indicators of lifestyle behaviours and do not fully capture all elements of these behaviours. For instance, our measure of unhealthy exercise did not incorporate the levels of exercise necessary to maximize its health benefits. While our measure has been used to identify persons who fall below the minimum recommended activity guidelines, it is only an approximation. Research into more precise exercise measures, such as calculating energy expenditure from frequency, duration, and metabolic values for all activities, can be done. However, this measure is only available in our national surveys from the mid-1990s. Also, using a BMI measure of 30+ is limited, because some persons who are overweight (e.g., BMI = 27–30) may also be at risk of various deleterious health effects, and some of those over 30 BMI may not be at risk. This is, in part, because BMI is not as accurate as some other body composition variables requiring physical or clinical measurement, such as skin fold measurement. With respect to smoking, we chose not to include previous smokers with current smokers, even though the former would still be exposed to some of cigarettes' deleterious effects on long-term health. To do so would have incorporated a layer of complexity to the cohort analyses that would have transcended the scope of this book. Overall, however, the lifestyle variables used in this research were constructed as conservative indicators; that is, they likely underestimate the unhealthy influence of one's lifestyle on health, and therefore the conclusions drawn from this research are likely reliable and accurate.

Second, the sample sizes of the surveys used in this research are not identical. In fact, they tended to increase over the 22-year period because of the growth in the population during this time, as well as the investment of greater resources by the government in order to collect health data with better accuracy for subgroups. Furthermore, the size of age-sex subgroups also changed because of population shifts. As a result, the sampling variability and error associated with the estimates provided here will not be the same across subgroups. Although this has implications when making comparisons across group and time, it should be noted that an error of this kind is likely to be nominal because the sizes of sub-samples are large. This was also established through the calculation of confidence intervals for all of the estimates, which proved to be extremely small. Thus, while some degree of sampling error was present when the comparisons were made, these are small and likely do not alter the findings.

Third, all of the measures (including chronic illnesses and health utilization) are based on self-reports. Although there is a relatively good correlation between self-reports and clinical reports, there is no doubt that there is some degree of measurement error. For example, it has been established that individuals generally overestimate their exercise levels and underestimate their body mass by approximately 10%. Again, this would tend to result in underestimations in this study. Fourth, population-based studies identify broad patterns and may overlook some of the more detailed trends in health behaviours and health status occurring among subgroups that are not included. Fifth, while comparisons of the baby boom generation, and earlier ones, included socio-economic, regional, and foreign-born gradients, it would be interesting as well to investigate other dimensions such as ethnic status variations. Finally, the healthy lifestyle indicators used in this research represent only a subset of preventive health behaviours requiring investigation.

Some of these limitations will be addressed once we collect enough data via the National Population Health Surveys, since these contain more detailed and standardized health measures on larger samples of individuals. However, these surveys only started in 1994/95 (repeated every two years), and the NPHS data will require several more years before it covers a long enough period to support age-period-cohort analyses. Furthermore, other types of research are certainly needed also to fill in these gaps; for example, multivariate analyses of longitudinal data to identify predictors of health factors, experimental design research to test interventions, and other related designs should prove useful.

Thus, there are many knowledge gaps left to fill with respect to population health – in particular, the ways in which health lifestyles are initiated, altered over time, and/or maintained. Opportunities for significant advancements in this field have presented themselves in a number of ways. There has been an infusion of new money into health research in recent years, in part due to the reorganization of the Medical Research Council and the National Health Research and Development Program into the newly evolved Canadian Institutes of Health Research (CIHR). Launched in 2000, CIHR was created with a mandate to excel, according to internationally accepted standards of scientific excellence, in the creation of new knowledge and its translation into improved health for Canadians, more effective health services and products, and a strengthened Canadian health care system (Bill C-13, 13 April 2000). Fundamental to this mandate is the translation of research into action with the support of effective partnerships and public engagement. In CIHR's *Blueprint for Health Research and Innovation* document, it is stated that in order to reach these goals, CIHR requires a sustained and up-front, multi-year funding commitment for growth in its budget from its current level of $620 million to $1 billion over the next four years (CIHR, 2003).

CIHR supports 13 research institutes with a wide range of innovative programs designed to encourage excellence and to catalyse multidisciplinary, collaborative research and research training: Aboriginal People's Health; Aging; Cancer; Circulatory and Respiratory Health; Gender; Genetics; Health Services and Policy; Human Development and Youth Health; Infection and Immunity; Musculoskeletal and Arthritis; Neurosciences, Mental Health, and Addictions; Nutrition, Metabolism and Diabetes; and Population and Public Health. Each of these institutes has identified research and action priorities and distributes grant funding in those target areas. For example, the Nutrition, Metabolism and Diabetes Institute has been funded for five years in the amount of $15 million to address issues of obesity and healthy body weight.

One of the limitations of the structure of the Canadian Institutes of Health is that they are organized around specific diseases, and grant funding tends to be targeted to those illnesses and their determinants. Joint initiatives across the institutes occur, but they need to be fostered. A multi-level approach that is directed towards several diseases, perhaps within a chronic disease model, and which addresses a constellation of risk factors simultaneously and interactively, may prove to be fruitful. This is not to say that several lifestyle behaviours are not being examined currently, but that there is likely greater potential for cross-fertilization among disease-based studies than what is being realized.

Furthermore, a universal, accessible, and primarily publicly funded health care system has been threatened because of a number of social, economic, and political shifts at the global, national, provincial, and regional levels. These include increasing privatization of services rooted in a growing corporate culture surrounding health care decisions, declining federal-provincial transfer payments, and shrinking citizen involvement and political will to make the necessary changes to the system. Contrary to popular opinion, our health care system is currently funded at approximately 70% to 30%, respectively, from public versus private sources. As noted in the famous Romonow Royal Commission on the Future of Health Care in Canada, increased funding and transformative change is paramount to sustain Medicare. Although a comprehensive discussion of health care reform in Canada is beyond the scope of this book, it is clear that reforms are needed, such as increased funding (e.g., a sustained rise in transfer payments to supplement the health deal signed in September 2004), expanded Canada Health Act coverage of programs and services (e.g., long-term care, a national comprehensive home care program, pharmacy/drug coverage, palliative care), and organization and standards of services (e.g., electronic patient records and health registry systems). However, it also needs to be recognized that health care is more than the provision of services once an individual is ill.

It is therefore vital to examine ways in which Canada's health care system can be utilized to promote healthy lifestyles. Currently, governments spend about $110 billion annually on Canada's health care system (CIHR, 2003), and it is clear that we need to tap fully into the ways in which this money can be used to achieve our health aims. Anticipated reforms to the Canadian system should investigate pathways to motivate people to maximize their involvement in their own health. Although there is movement in this direction among some individuals, as evidenced in the increase in self-management of chronic illness, and the expanded use of complementary and alternative medicine (Wister, Chittenden, McCoy, Wilson, Allen, and Wong, 2002), there can be a lot more to learn from the health care systems of other countries. For example, while there are deficiencies in the group insurance system in the United States, this system offers some positive lessons as well. Health insurance systems that use direct financial incentives (i.e., lower insurance rates) for members who can improve and/or maintain lifestyle risk factors may prove to be effective. There have also been developments in computerized health registries (and disease registries) that can be used to monitor changes in lifestyle and clinical risk factors, in order to be more proactive in the prevention of disease and the maintenance of health and well-being. Such changes might be adapted to our health care system without compromizing the essential components of the Canada Health Act or Medicare. The Canadian system undoubtedly will adapt and reform in the coming years, and in doing so may benefit from cross-national comparative studies that in turn may reveal innovative ways to make our system more proactive in promoting health. However, health care reform must mean more than simply reducing number of beds and closing hospitals in order to balance budgets, or, conversely, shortening waiting times for surgery.

Finally, while researchers are now beginning to recognize the potential of multidisciplinary research, many hurdles need to be crossed in order to move us to the next level. As noted in earlier chapters, a new paradigm has been articulated in response to the recent era of what has been called 'eco-epidemiology' (McMichael, 1999; Susser and Susser, 1996a, 1996b). The analytical approach, termed the Chinese Boxes, identifies determinants and outcomes at different levels of organization: within and between contexts (using new information systems), and in depth (using new biological systems). It therefore acknowledges the inherent connectedness among domains such as populations, communities, families, single individuals, and individual biological systems. It also emphasises the salience of specifying the underlying etiology of health and illness. The principal idea is that we must move beyond proximate causes of health status to examine and link factors in a full causal chain. This type of research requires innovation at all levels, including funding, theoretical development, and basic and applied research.

Conclusion and Future Scenarios

We now have uncovered a number of new insights into patterns of healthy and unhealthy lifestyles of Canadians, with a focus on baby boomers as they age. Our investigations were directed by Riley's (1993) Social Change Model, which points our attention towards the interplay of individual and structural factors through the conceptions of age stratification, life course, and cohort analysis. Key questions guiding this book included (1) Are the baby boomers healthier or unhealthier than previous generations? and (2) What are the implications of these patterns for the Canadian health care system? Current knowledge in this field has been sparse and fraught with stereotypical images rather than fact. Some researchers describe 'boomers' as individuals who are in better health and financially better off than prior generations, whereas others maintain that they are prone to unhealthy lifestyles and chronic illness, and indeed will break the public purse when they become the 'elderly of tomorrow.' These questions are fundamental to the future of Canadian society, given that the baby boom generation comprises approximately one-third of the population, and, moreover, are moving up the age escalator to the top floors. Our answers to these questions appear to be considerably more complex than previously thought.

Compared to the previous generation, baby boomers have reduced their levels of what we have termed unhealthy exercise, as well as smoking and heavy drinking. However, obesity is on an accelerated progression, and may outstrip gains associated with these other major health behaviours – indeed, it is not surprising that obesity is being given the label 'the new tobacco.' And yet, there is some evidence that we may have reached the obesity threshold, and possibly the beginning signs of a reversal in this trend. Still, overall it is probably more accurate to conclude that baby boomers are different than the previous generation in terms of healthy lifestyles, rather than better or worse. Furthermore, the nature of chronic illness facing the baby boomers is also changing shape compared to the earlier generation. Although diabetes, respiratory diseases, and dementia appear to be on the rise, and several other diseases are on the decline, coronary heart disease and cancer likely will remain the most common chronic illness for baby boomers. Given that there are limits to the degree to which morbidity can be compressed near the end of life, a greater issue for the baby boomers may relate to the types, severity, and timing of chronic illnesses that they will likely experience, rather than the 'pandemic of chronic illness' as espoused by Dychtwald (1997). Thus, there is both good and bad news concerning how we are aging as a nation, but it appears that time is still on our side in our efforts to abandon deleterious health and lifestyle patterns and to maintain the beneficial ones.

We have also learned that healthy lifestyles are fundamental to the health of individuals and populations. Yet, these lifestyles involve multifaceted and sometimes ephemeral behaviours that require delineation and contextualization within a complex set of micro-meso-macro processes. Our investigation of lifestyle patterns revealed a number of anomalies, as well; in particular, that there is a paradox in the concurrent trends of improving levels of exercise and an obesity epidemic that has traversed virtually every group in society over the last few decades. In order to explain this apparent disconnect in lifestyle trends, changes in leisure-time physical activity, work-related physical activity, eating habits, fast food super-sizing, and environmental factors influencing healthy lifestyles were investigated not only for baby boomers, but for the general population as well. The finger seems to be pointing at food consumption, yet Canadians also should not become complacent about their level of physical activity.

This work has been positioned within a number of debates regarding health care reform. It has addressed several questions and issues that have attracted the attention of researchers, policy-makers, and health care organizations; for example, how will the baby boomers influence future patterns of health utilization? The results of our analyses of population health have established that there have been increases in some chronic illnesses and declines in others. For this reason, it may be vital to our health care system that it adapt to a rapidly changing illness landscape. A formula for the future must include not only factors that influence the demand for services, such as growth in the health sector, but also those that shape the supply side, such as the prevalence of poor health behaviours and illness as well as knowledge and expectations, which appear to be higher among the baby boomers. We must also consider interrelationships among both supply and demand components of the population health formula.

The fact that we spend approximately $110 billion per year on a health care system in which very few resources are devoted to understanding the etiology and mutability of healthy lifestyles suggests that it may be time for a new direction. A health care system is more than the funding and organization of health services – it is a model of how people can maximize health. There is no reason why Canada should not be a leader in health care as well as in population health. Canadians are known around the world for their high standard of living, joy of sports, and peacekeeping policies. To add healthy lifestyles to this list will require an expansion of our current national identity. But this will only occur if we can meet the challenge of committing to a significant progression in the development and reinforcement of healthy behaviours, those that will comprise our daily routines and ultimately shape our health trajectories for the better as we pass through life.

Finally, this book has reinforced the idea that making predictions about what the baby boomers will be like when they are old, and what this will mean for them and for society, is like hitting a moving target. Future scenarios that are based on simple linear projections, statements of crises, or apocalyptic notions will invariably be proven wrong. That is not to say that the baby boomers should be ignored or that they will not pose new challenges and issues. Indeed, it appears that we can anticipate a rising prevalence of obesity, diabetes, dementia, and certain cancers; an older population with greater health knowledge and expectations of the health care system; and substantial demand for various health-related services and support systems due to the sheer numbers of baby boomers, as our population ages. Yet, to contend that baby boomers will break the health care or pension systems, or that they will cause a 'pandemic of chronic illness,' creates a debate that invariably leads us away from what is really important: detailing the complexities of the health dynamics of the baby boomers as they age. The only conclusion of certainty is that significant investment into further basic and applied research, as well as health promotion and population health initiatives, is not only warranted, but imperative, if we are to improve the health of the nation while adapting to the nuances of population aging in the new millennium.

Appendix

Table A8.1
Percentage of Canadian Population Aged 35–54 Who Are Regular Smokers,
1978/79–2000/01

| | Age Group | | | | | |
| | 35–44 | | 45–54 | | 35–54 | |
Survey	N	%	N	%	N	%
1978/79 CHS	960,051	43.8	855,212	43.7	1,815,262	43.8
1985 HPS	1,146,425	32.5	840,782	33.4	1,987,207	32.8
1990 HPS	1,367,022	33.0	780,025	28.1	2,150,040	31.0
1994/95 NPHS	1,464,224	30.1	933,835	26.7	2,398,059	28.7
2000/01 CCHS	1,438,018	27.2	1,101,670	24.9	2,539,688	26.1

Note: Numbers are weighted to the population.

Table A8.2
Percentage of Canadian Population Aged 35–54 Who Are Sedentary or Infrequent
Exercisers*, 1978/79–2000/01

| | Age Group | | | | | |
| | 35–44 | | 45–54 | | 35–54 | |
Survey	N	%	N	%	N	%
1978/79 CHS	1,356,902	64.6	1,293,313	68.6	2,650,215	66.5
1985 HPS	1,781,228	50.5	1,269,983	50.4	3,051,211	50.4
1990 HPS	2,343,017	56.6	1,498,509	53.4	3,841,526	55.3
1994/95 NPHS	2,281,875	46.9	1,665,969	47.5	3,947,844	47.2
2000/01 CCHS	2,085,998	39.4	1,732,085	39.2	3,818,083	39.3

Note: Numbers are weighted to the population.
*Sedentary/infrequent exerciser = 15 min. of physical activity <3X per week.

Table A8.3
Percentage of Canadian Population Aged 35–54 Who Are Obese (BMI 30+),
1985–2000/01*

| Survey | Age Group | | | | | |
| | 35–44 | | 45–54 | | 35–54 | |
	N	%	N	%	N	%
1985 HPS	248,684	7.0	244,513	9.7	493,198	8.2
1990 HPS	415,417	10.0	342,810	12.2	758,227	10.9
1994/95 NPHS	609,750	12.5	572,554	16.3	1,182,304	14.1
2000/01 CCHS	779,708	14.7	795,188	18.0	1,574,896	16.2

Note: Numbers are weighted to the population.
*Since BMI was collected only for a sub-sample composed of about 20% of the
1978/79 CHS sample, the population estimates are unreliable and have been omitted.

Table A8.4
Percentage of Canadian Population Aged 35–54 Who Are Heavy Drinkers*,
1978/79–2000/01

| Survey | Age Group | | | | | |
| | 35–44 | | 45–54 | | 35–54 | |
	N	%	N	%	N	%
1978/79 CHS	294,764	14.1	249,838	13.5	544,602	13.8
1985 HPS**	340,045	9.6	204,462	8.1	544,507	9.0
1990 HPS	301,674	7.3	232,792	8.3	534,465	7.7
1994/95 NPHS	319,089	6.6	225,264	6.4	544,353	6.5
2000/01 CCHS	319,453	6.0	289,676	6.6	609,130	6.3

Note: Numbers are weighted to the population.
*Heavy drinker = 14+ drinks/week for males and 12+ drinks/week for females.
**The midpoint of categories representing a range of number of drinks consumed per
week was used as an estimate of drinking behaviour for the 1985 HPS data; since the
highest category was 12+ drinks, these calculations may underestimate the % of heavy
drinkers for this year.

Table A8.5
Percentage of Canadian Population Aged 35–54 with a Chronic Condition,
1978/79–2000/01*

| Survey | Age Group | | | | | |
| | 35–44 | | 45–54 | | 35–54 | |
	N	%	N	%	N	%
1978/79 CHS	1,241,613	46.6	1,465,783	60.0	2,707,396	53.0
1994/95 NPHS	2,335,856	48.0	1,999,448	57.1	4,335,304	51.8
1998/99 NPHS	2,946,192	54.4	2,529,733	63.7	5,475,927	58.3
2000/01 CCHS	3,158,492	60.1	2,934,568	66.8	6,093,060	63.1

Note: Numbers are weighted to the population.
*1985 and 1990 data are not available for chronic conditions.

Table A8.6
Percentage of Canadian Population Aged 35–54 with Hypertension, 1978/79–2000/01*

| Survey | Age Group | | | | | |
| | 05–44 | | 45–54 | | 35–54 | |
	N	%	N	%	N	%
1978/79 CHS	105,557	4.0	308,927	12.7	414,483	8.1
1994/95 NPHS	202,803	4.2	350,870	10.0	553,673	6.6
1998/99 NPHS	267,752	4.9	441,567	11.1	709,320	7.5
2000/01 CCHS	313,528	5.9	627,170	14.2	940,698	9.7

Note: Numbers are weighted to the population.
*1985 and 1990 data are not available for chronic conditions.

Table A8.7
Percentage of Canadian Population Aged 35–54 with Arthritis, 1978/79–2000/01*

| Survey | Age Group | | | | | |
| | 35–44 | | 45–54 | | 35–54 | |
	N	%	N	%	N	%
1978/79 CHS	227,085	8.5	465,344	19.1	692,429	13.6
1994/95 NPHS	332,391	6.8	487,504	13.9	819,894	9.8
1998/99 NPHS	459,390	8.5	686,618	17.2	1,146,008	12.2
2000/01 CCHS	466,348	8.8	755,224	17.1	1,221,571	12.6

Note: Numbers are weighted to the population.
*1985 and 1990 data are not available for chronic conditions.

Table A8.8
Percentage of Canadian Population Aged 35–54 with Diabetes, 1978/79–2000/01*

| | Age Group | | | | | |
| | 35–44 | | 45–54 | | 35–54 | |
Survey	N	%	N	%	N	%
1978/79 CHS	28,897	1.1	55,635	2.3	84,532	1.7
1994/95 NPHS	72,925	1.5	85,636	2.4	158,561	1.9
1998/99 NPHS	85,944	1.6	133,925	3.4	219,870	2.3
2000/01 CCHS	102,558	1.9	189,641	4.3	292,199	3.0

Note: Numbers are weighted to the population.
*1985 and 1990 data are not available for chronic conditions.

Table A8.9
Percentage of Canadian Population Aged 35–54 Reporting 3+ Doctor Visits in the Past 12 Months, 1978/79–2000/01*

| | Age Group | | | | | |
| | 35–44 | | 45–54 | | 35–54 | |
Survey	N	%	N	%	N	%
1978/79 CHS	826,994	31.3	863,502	35.6	1,690,496	33.3
1994/95 NPHS	2,290,252	47.1	1,761,758	50.4	4,052,010	48.5
1998/99 NPHS	2,561,855	47.3	2,030,727	51.0	4,592,582	48.9
2000/01 CCHS	2,478,957	46.9	2,319,172	52.6	4,798,128	49.5

Note: Numbers are weighted to the population.
*1985 and 1990 data are not available for doctors visits.

Table A9.1
Percentage of Canadian Population Aged 35–54 Who Are Regular Smokers by Level of
Education, 1978/79–2000/01

Survey year	≤HS grad. N	%	>HS grad. N	%	Group % diff.[1]	Relative % diff.[2]
1978/79	1,461,409	47.9	342,830	31.9	−16.0	−33.4
1985	1,410,182	26.3	438,787	24.2	−2.1	−8.0
1990	1,391,102	37.7	709,234	23.0	−14.7	−39.0
1994/95	1,104,898	35.7	1,289,300	24.5	−11.2	−31.4
2000/01	1,245,102	34.6	1,258,057	20.9	−13.7	−39.6

Note: Numbers are weighted to the population.
1. Group % difference is calculated as: high education % minus low education % for
each survey year.
2. Relative % difference is calculated as: high education % minus low education %
divided by low education %.

Table A9.2
Percentage of Canadian Population Aged 35–54 Who Are Sedentary or Infrequent
Exercisers* by Level of Education, 1978/79–2000/01

Survey year	≤HS grad. N	%	>HS grad. N	%	Group % diff.[1]	Relative % diff.[2]
1978/79	202,257	69.3	614,802	58.6	−10.7	−15.4
1985	2,822,111	53.3	758,808	41.9	−11.4	−21.4
1990	2,064,262	56.1	1,682,835	54.7	−1.4	−2.5
1994/95	1,575,498	53.2	2,364,267	47.2	−6.0	−11.3
2000/01	1,616,258	48.6	2,160,861	38.2	−10.4	−21.4

Note: Numbers are weighted to the population.
*Sedentary/infrequent exerciser = 15 min. of physical activity <3X per week.
1. Group % difference is calculated as: high education % minus low education % for
each survey year.
2. Relative % difference is calculated as: high education % minus low education %
divided by low education %.

Table A9.3
Percentage of Canadian Population Aged 35–54 Who Are Obese (BMI 30+) by Level of Education, 1985–2000/01*

Survey year	≤HS grad.		>HS grad.		Group % diff.[1]	Relative % diff.[2]
	N	%	N	%		
1985	469,603	8.8	103,573	5.8	−3.0	−34.0
1990	476,927	13.0	263,346	8.6	−4.4	−33.8
1994/95	469,673	15.4	711,237	13.8	−1.6	−10.4
2000/01	667,727	19.0	895,009	15.2	−3.8	−20.0

Note: Numbers are weighted to the population.
*Since BMI was collected only for a sub-sample composed of about 20% of the 1978/79 CHS sample, the population estimates are unreliable and have been omitted.
1. Group % difference is calculated as: high education % minus low education % for each survey year.
2. Relative % difference is calculated as: high education % minus low education % divided by low education %.

Table A9.4
Percentage of Canadian Population Aged 35–54 Who Are Heavy Drinkers* by Level of Education, 1978/79–2000/01

Survey year	≤HS grad.		>HS grad.		Group % diff.[1]	Relative % diff.[2]
	N	%	N	%		
1978/79	391,000	13.6	151,681	14.6	1.0	7.3
1985	332,905	6.3	173,076	9.6	3.3	52.4
1990	275,856	7.5	248,608	8.1	0.6	8.0
1994/95	197,599	6.4	345,829	6.6	0.2	3.1
2000/01	235,393	6.6	368,025	6.2	−0.4	−6.1

Note: Numbers are weighted to the population.
*'Heavy drinker' is defined as 14+ drinks/week for males and 12+ drinks/week for females.
**The midpoint of categories representing a range of number of drinks consumed per week was used as an estimate of drinking behaviour for the 1985 HPS data; as the highest category was 12+ drinks, these calculations may underestimate the % of heavy drinkers for this year.
1. Group % difference is calculated as: high education % minus low education % for each survey year.
2. Relative % difference is calculated as: high education % minus low education % divided by low education %.

Table A9.5
Percentage of Canadian Population Aged 35–54 Who Are Regular
Smokers by Income Level*, 1978/79–2000/01

Survey year	Low income** N	%	High income** N	%	Group % diff.[1]	Relative % diff.[2]
1978/79	357,224	51.4	1,339,757	42.1	−9.3	−18.1
1985	396,764	40.0	1,104,309	32.4	−7.6	−19.0
1990	594,298	43.1	1,346,771	27.5	−15.6	−36.2
1994/95	773,011	40.1	1,536,439	25.4	−14.7	−36.7
2000/01	615,880	39.6	1,748,024	23.8	−15.8	−39.9

Note: Numbers are weighted to the population.
*Total yearly household income.
**Income levels are split at median based on 2000 real dollar conversions. The following median values were used: 1978/79 = $14,000; 1985 = $23,000; 1990, 1994/95 & 2000/01= $30,000.
1. Group % difference is calculated as: high income % minus low income % for each survey year.
2. Relative % difference is calculated as: high income % minus low income % divided by low income %.

Table A9.6
Percentage of Canadian Population Aged 35–54 Who Are Sedentary or Infrequent
Exercisers° by Income Level*, 1978/79–2000/01

Survey year	Low income** N	%	High income** N	%	Group % diff.[1]	Relative % diff.[2]
1978/79	454,043	68.6	2,021,257	65.9	−2.7	−3.9
1985	491,635	49.9	1,696,457	49.9	0	0
1990	788,099	57.3	2,713,788	55.5	−1.8	−3.1
1994/95	1,003,278	53.9	2,771,425	48.0	−5.9	−10.9
2000/01	743,837	50.9	2,770,014	40.1	−10.8	−21.2

Note: Numbers are weighted to the population.
°Sedentary/Infrequent exerciser = 15 min. of physical activity <3X per week.
*Total yearly household income.
**Income levels are split at median based on 2000 real dollar conversions. The following median values were used: 1978/79 = $14,000; 1985 = $23,000; 1990, 1994/95 & 2000/01 = $30,000.
1. Group % difference is calculated as: high income % minus low income % for each survey year.
2. Relative % difference is calculated as: high income % minus low income % divided by low income %.

Table A9.7

Percentage of Canadian Population Aged 35–54 Who Are Obese (BMI = 30+) by Income Level*, 1985–2000/01°

Survey year	Low income** N	%	High income** N	%	Group % diff.[1]	Relative % diff.[2]
1985	79,031	8.0	273,289	8.2	0.2	2.5
1990	199,999	14.7	502,431	10.3	−4.4	−29.9
1994/95	314,483	16.6	814,722	13.6	−3.0	−18.1
2000/01	277,612	18.3	1,196,646	16.5	−1.8	−9.8

Note: Numbers are weighted to the population.
°Since BMI was collected only for a sub-sample composed of about 20% of the 1978/79 CHS sample, the population estimates are unreliable and have been omitted.
*Total yearly household income.
**Income levels are split at median based on 2000 real dollar conversions. The following median values were used: 1978/79 = $14,000; 1985 = $23,000; 1990, 1994/95 & 2000/01 = $30,000.
1. Group % difference is calculated as: high income % minus low income % for each survey year.
2. Relative % difference is calculated as: high income % minus low income % divided by low income %.

Table A9.8

Percentage of Canadian Population Aged 35–54 Who Are Heavy Drinkers° by Income Level*, 1978/79–2000/01

Survey year	Low income** N	%	High income** N	%	Group % diff.[1]	Relative % diff.[2]
1978/79	63,392	9.9	455,422	15.0	5.1	51.5
1985	71,822	7.3	377,297	11.2	3.9	53.4
1990	51,146	3.7	442,334	9.1	5.4	145.9
1994/95	110,333	5.7	405,024	6.7	1.0	17.5
2000/01	79,484	5.1	498,025	6.8	1.7	33.3

Note: Numbers are weighted to the population.
°'Heavy drinker' is defined as 14+ drinks/week for males and 12+ drinks/week for females.
*Total yearly household income.
**Income levels are split at median based on 2000 real dollar conversions. The following median values were used: 1978/79 = $14,000; 1985 = $23,000; 1990, 1994/95 & 2000/01 = $30,000.
1. Group % difference is calculated as: high income % minus low income % for each survey year.
2. Relative % difference is calculated as: high income % minus low income % divided by low income %.

Table A9.9
Percentage of Canadian Population Aged 35–54 Who Are Regular Smokers by Region, 1978/79–2000/01

Survey year	Atlantic		Quebec		Ontario		Prairies		BC	
	N	%	N	%	N	%	N	%	N	%
1978/79	153,259	47.1	590,924	43.7	581,756	39.4	293,505	44.4	195,818	41.6
1985	222,564	30.1	746,249	33.6	834,178	26.7	354,062	25.8	241,011	23.7
1990	192,432	33.0	673,073	36.4	737,316	28.9	341,539	30.6	212,588	25.3
1994/95	212,505	32.0	770,862	35.3	812,560	26.0	355,895	27.0	246,237	22.9
2000/01	216,030	29.1	721,101	30.5	918,854	24.4	423,249	27.3	249,365	20.0

Note: Numbers are weighted to the population.

Table A9.10
Percentage of Canadian Population Aged 35–54 Who Are Sedentary or Infrequent Exercisers* by Region, 1978/79–2000/01

Survey year	Atlantic		Quebec		Ontario		Prairies		BC	
	N	%	N	%	N	%	N	%	N	%
1978/79	235,882	76.9	810,828	67.3	904,318	64.6	438,115	68.0	261,073	60.7
1985	355,040	48.9	1,255,636	56.7	1,560,763	50.1	606,406	44.4	425,768	42.1
1990	310,930	53.8	1,147,776	62.0	1,383,420	54.3	571,919	51.8	427,481	51.1
1994/95	356,419	56.1	1,149,883	54.8	1,519,410	50.9	547,296	44.2	374,836	36.7
2000/01	305,431	43.9	1,071,339	47.8	1,476,993	41.6	585,089	40.8	368,923	33.1

Note: Numbers are weighted to the population.
*Sedentary/Infrequent exerciser = 15 min. of physical activity <3X per week.

Table A9.11
Percentage of Canadian Population Aged 35–54 Who Are Obese (BMI 30+) by Region, 1985–2000/01*

Survey year	Atlantic		Quebec		Ontario		Prairies		BC	
	N	%	N	%	N	%	N	%	N	%
1985	74,318	10.2	157,119	7.2	197,146	6.4	153,349	11.3	62,679	6.2
1990	83,036	14.4	130,731	7.1	307,441	12.2	139,523	12.6	97,497	11.8
1994/95	124,237	19.0	233,653	10.8	491,792	16.0	213,999	16.7	118,623	11.1
2000/01	163,382	22.5	320,066	13.7	630,403	17.1	292,795	19.3	161,665	13.3

Note: Numbers are weighted to the population.
*Since BMI was collected only for a sub-sample composed of about 20% of the 1978/79 CHS sample, the population estimates are unreliable and have been omitted.

Table A9.12
Percentage of Canadian Population Aged 35–54 Who Are Heavy Drinkers* by Region, 1978/79–2000/01

Survey year	Atlantic		Quebec		Ontario		Prairies		BC	
	N	%	N	%	N	%	N	%	N	%
1978/79	26,267	8.8	120,009	10.5	209,749	14.9	105,387	16.5	83,190	18.2
1985**	26,518	3.6	135,096	6.1	315,649	10.2	68,624	5.0	118,648	11.8
1990	31,384	5.4	145,088	7.8	232,348	9.2	77,806	7.0	47,839	5.7
1994/95	37,262	5.6	119,900	5.6	235,544	7.6	76,600	5.8	75,046	7.0
2000/01	41,700	5.6	170,298	7.2	233,460	6.2	87,040	5.6	74,731	6.1

Note: Numbers are weighted to the population.

*'Heavy drinker' is defined as 14+ drinks/week for males and 12+ drinks/week for females.

**The midpoint of categories representing a range of number of drinks consumed per week was used as an estimate of drinking behaviour for the 1985 HPS data; as the highest category was 12+ drinks, these calculations may underestimate the % of heavy drinkers for this year.

Table A9.13
Percentage of Canadian Population Aged 35–54 Who Are Regular Smokers by
Foreign-Born Status, 1978/79–2000/01*

| | Foreign-Born | | Canadian-Born | |
Survey year	N	%	N	%
1978/79	347,040	35.0	1,464,340	46.5
1994/95	288,620	15.7	2,091,679	32.4
1998/99	306,099	14.1	2,223,181	30.8
2000/01	343,426	15.6	2,181,358	29.3

Note: Numbers are weighted to the population.
*Place of birth was not collected for the 1985 and 1990 HPS.

Table A9.14
Percentage of Canadian Population Aged 35–54 Who Are Sedentary or Infrequent
Exercisers* by Foreign-Born Status, 1978/79–2000/01**

| | Foreign-Born | | Canadian-Born | |
Survey year	N	%	N	%
1978/79	627,763	65.1	2,014,555	66.9
1994/95	915,176	53.4	3,015,503	48.5
1998/99	932,250	44.4	2,604,396	36.6
2000/01	992,853	49.9	2,797,914	39.9

Note: Numbers are weighted to the population.
*Sedentary/Infrequent exerciser = 15 min. of physical activity <3X per week.
**Place of birth was not collected for the 1985 and 1990 HPS.

Table A9.15
Percentage of Canadian Population Aged 35–54 who are Obese (BMI 30+) by
Foreign-born Status, 1994/95–2000/01*

Survey year	Foreign-Born		Canadian-Born	
	N	%	N	%
1994/95	186,791	10.3	992,201	15.6
1998/99	249,106	11.6	1,264,073	17.8
2000/01	263,316	12.2	1,304,872	17.9

Note: Numbers are weighted to the population.
*Since BMI was collected only for a sub-sample composed of about 20% of the 1978/79
CHS sample, the population estimates are unreliable and have been omitted; place of
birth was not collected for the 1985 and 1990 HPS.

Table A9.16
Percentage of Canadian Population Aged 35–54 Who Are Heavy Drinkers* by
Foreign-born Status, 1978/79–2000/01**

Survey year	Foreign-Born		Canadian-Born	
	N	%	N	%
1978/79	1,29,301	13.5	415,020	14.0
1994/95	105,326	5.8	436,946	6.8
1998/99	157,720	7.2	593,128	8.2
2000/01	73,254	3.3	533,685	7.2

Note: Numbers are weighted to the population.
*'Heavy drinker' is defined as 14+ drinks/week for males and 12+ drinks/week for
females.
**Place of birth was not collected for the 1985 and 1990 HPS.

Figure A1 Percentage of Canadian Population Regular Smokers by 5-Year Age Groups, Males and Females, 1978/79

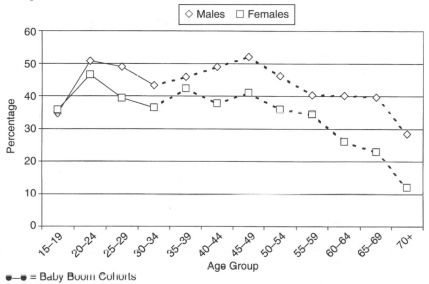

●—● = Baby Boom Cohorts

Figure A2 Percentage of Canadian Population Regular Smokers by 5-Year Age Groups, Males and Females, 1985*

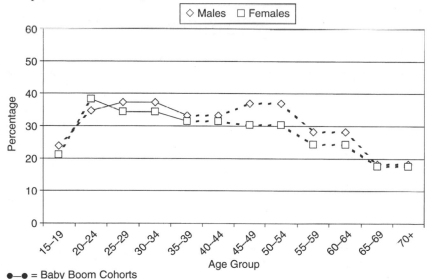

●—● = Baby Boom Cohorts

*To smooth out variation due to sampling error, average smoking rates for 10-year age groups, starting with age 25, were calculated and applied to 5-year age groups.

Figure A3 Percentage of Canadian Population Regular Smokers by 5-Year Age Groups, Males and Females, 1990

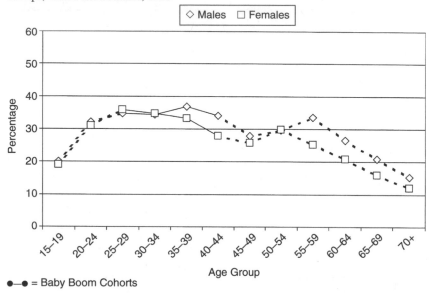

●—● = Baby Boom Cohorts

Figure A4 Percentage of Canadian Population Regular Smokers by 5-Year Age Groups, Males and Females, 1994/95

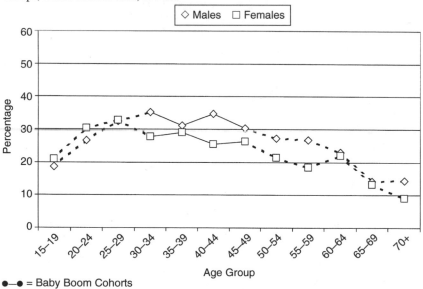

●—● = Baby Boom Cohorts

Figure A5 Percentage of Canadian Population Regular Smokers by 5-Year Age
Groups, Males and Females, 2000/01

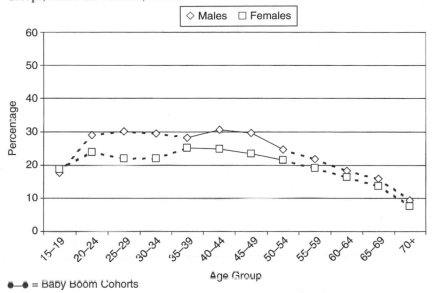

●—● = Baby Boom Cohorts

Figure A6 Percentage of Canadian Population Sedentary or Infrequent Exercisers*
by 5-Year Age Groups, Males and Females, 1978/79

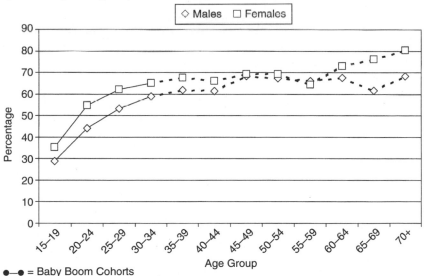

●—● = Baby Boom Cohorts
*15 min. of physical activity <3X per week.

Figure A7 Percentage of Canadian Population Sedentary or Infrequent Exercisers* by 5-Year Age Groups, Males and Females, 1985

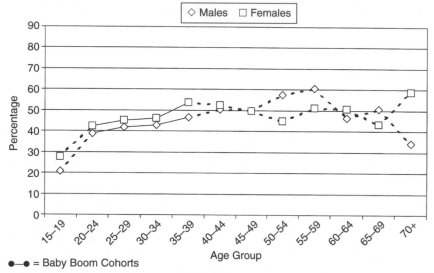

●—● = Baby Boom Cohorts

*15 min. of physical activity <3X per week.

Figure A8 Percentage of Canadian Population Sedentary or Infrequent Exercisers* by 5-Year Age Groups, Males and Females, 1990

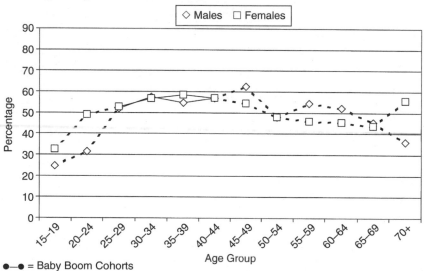

●—● = Baby Boom Cohorts

*15 min. of physical activity <3X per week.

Figure A9 Percentage of Canadian Population Sedentary or Infrequent Exercisers* by 5-Year Age Groups, Males and Females, 1994/95

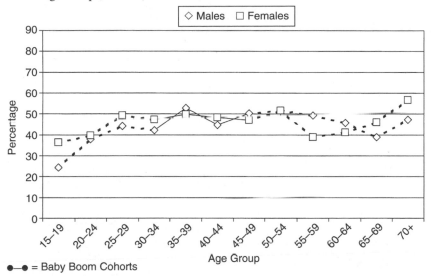

●—● = Baby Boom Cohorts

*15 min. of physical activity <3X per week.

Figure A10 Percentage of Canadian Population Sedentary or Infrequent Exercisers* by 5-Year Age Groups, Males and Females, 2000/01

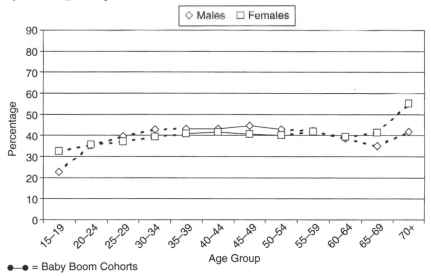

●—● = Baby Boom Cohorts

*15 min. of physical activity <3X per week.

Figure A11 Percentage of Canadian Population Obese (BMI 30+) by 5-Year Age Groups, Males and Females, 1985

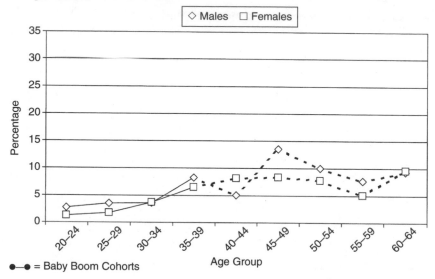

●—● = Baby Boom Cohorts

Figure A12 Percentage of Canadian Population Obese (BMI 30+) by 5-Year Age Groups, Males and Females, 1990

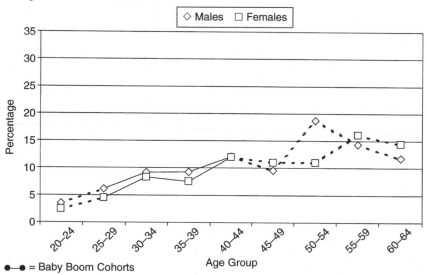

●—● = Baby Boom Cohorts

Figure A13 Percentage of Canadian Population Obese (BMI 30+) by 5-Year Age
Groups, Males and Females, 1994/95

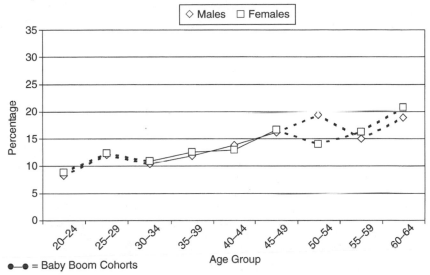

●—● = Baby Boom Cohorts

Figure A14 Percentage of Canadian Population Obese (BMI 30+) by 5-Year Age
Groups, Males and Females, 2000/01

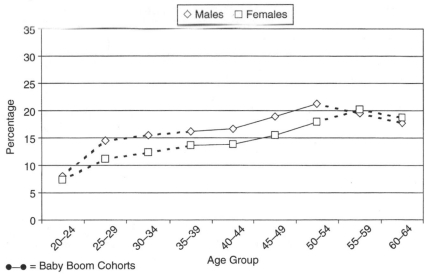

●—● = Baby Boom Cohorts

Figure A15 Percentage of Canadian Population Heavy Drinkers* by 5-Year Age Groups, Males and Females, 1978/79

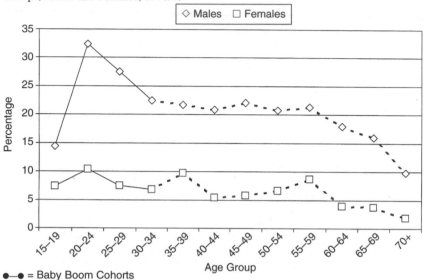

●—● = Baby Boom Cohorts
*Males = 14+ drinks/week; females = 12+ drinks/week.

Figure A16 Percentage of Canadian Population Heavy Drinkers* by 5-Year Age Groups, Males and Females, 1985**

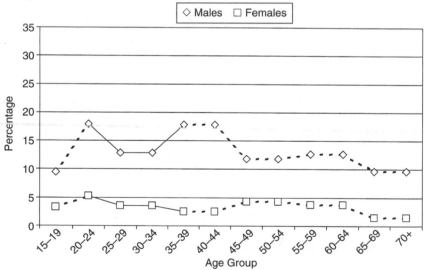

●—● = Baby Boom Cohorts
*Males = 14+ drinks/week; females = 12+ drinks/week.
**To smooth out variation due to sampling error, average smoking rates for 10-year age groups, starting with age 25, were calculated and applied to 5-year age groups.

Figure A17 Percentage of Canadian Population Heavy Drinkers* by 5-Year Age
Groups, Males and Females, 1990

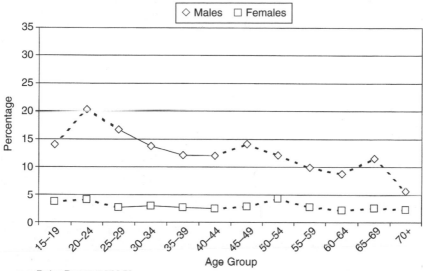

●—● = Baby Boom Cohorts

*Males = 14+ drinks/week; females = 12+ drinks/week.

Figure A18 Percentage of Canadian Population Heavy Drinkers* by 5-Year Age
Groups, Males and Females, 1994/95

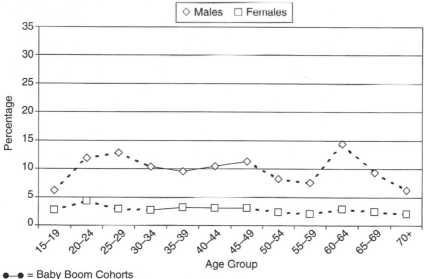

●—● = Baby Boom Cohorts

*Males = 14+ drinks/week; females = 12+ drinks/week.

Figure A19 Percentage of Canadian Population Heavy Drinkers* by 5-Year Age Groups, Males and Females, 2000/01

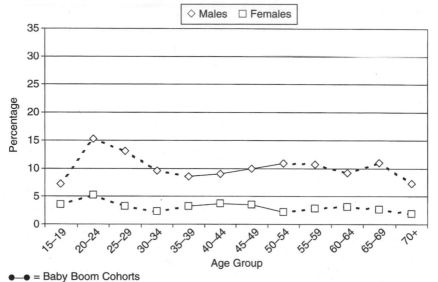

●—● = Baby Boom Cohorts

*Males = 14+ drinks/week; females = 12+ drinks/week.

References

Alain, B. 1999. The eating habits of Canadians. *Insights* 3(2):5–7.

American Council on Science and Health. 1999. *Environmental tobacco smoke: Health risk or health hype?* New York: American Council on Science and Health.

Antonovsky, A. 1967. Social class, life expectancy and overall mortality. *The Milbank Quarterly* 45:31–73.

Antonovsky, A. 1979. *Health, stress, and coping.* San Francisco: Jossey-Bass.

Andrews, F. 1988. *Alcohol use. Canada's health promotion survey: Technical report.* Cat. II39–119/1988E. Ottawa: Minister of Supply and Services.

Bandura, A. 1977. Self-efficacy: Toward a unifying theory of behavioral change. *Psychology Review* 84:191–215.

Barer, M., R. Evans, and C. Hertzman,. 1995. Avalanche or glacier? Health care and the demographic rhetoric. *Canadian Journal on Aging* 14(2):193–224.

Béland, Y. 2002. Canadian community health survey – Methodological overview. *Health Reports* 13:9–14.

Berkman, L.F. 1984. Assessing the physical health effects of social networks and social support in the elderly. *Journal of the American Geriatrics Society* 31(12): 743–749.

Berkman, L.F., and I. Kawachi. 2000. *Social epidemiology.* New York: Oxford University Press.

Berkman, L., and S. Syme. 1979. Social networks, host resistance, and mortality: A nine-year follow-up study of Alameda County residents. *American Journal of Epidemiology* 109: 186–204.

Best, A., D. Stokols, L. Green, S. Leischow, B. Holmes, and K. Buchholz. 2003. An integrative framework for community partnering to translate theory into effective health promotion strategy. *American Journal of Health Promotion* 18(2):168–176.

Binkley, J., J. Eales, and M. Jekanowski. 2000. The relation between dietary change and rising U.S. obesity. *International Journal of Obesity* 24:1032–1039.

Black, C., N. Roos, B. Havens, and L. MacWilliam. 1995. Rising use of physician services by the elderly: The contribution of morbidity. *Canadian Journal on Aging* 14(2):225–244.

Blanchette, P., and V. Valcour. 1998. Health and aging among baby boomers. *Generations* 22(1):76–80.

Boyd, M. and M. Vickers. 2000. 100 years of immigration in Canada. *Canadian Social Trends* 58(Autumn):2–12.

Cairney, J., and T. Wade. 1998. Correlates of body weight in the 1994 National Population Health Survey. *International Journal of Obesity* 22:584–591.

Canadian Association of Cardiac Rehabilitation. 1999. *Canadian guidelines for cardiac rehabilitation and cardiovascular disease prevention.* Winnipeg: Canadian Association of Cardiac Rehabilitation.

Canadian Fitness and Lifestyle Research Institute. 1998. *Progress in prevention bulletin.* Ottawa: Canadian Fitness and Lifestyle Research Institute.

Canadian Population Health Initiative. 2004. *Improving the Health of Canadians.* Ottawa: Canadian Institute for Health Information.

Canadian Study of Health and Aging Working Group. 1994. Canadian Study of Health and Aging: Study methods and prevalence of dementia. *Journal of the Canadian Medical Association* 150(6):899–914.

Carrière, Y., and J. Légaré. 1993. Vieillissement démographique et institutionnalisation des personnes âgées: Des projections nuancées pour le Québec. *Cahiers Québécois de Démographie* 22(1):63–92.

Carrière, Y., and L. Pelletier. 1995. Factors underlying the institutionalization of elderly persons in Canada. *Journal of Gerontology: Social Sciences* 50B(3):S164–S172.

Centers for Disease Control. 1996. *Behavioral Risk Factor Surveillance System, Series 1, No.1, 1984–1995.* [CD-ROM]. Atlanta: Centers for Disease Control.

Centers for Disease Control. 2000. Cigarette smoking-related mortality.' http://www.cdc.gov/tobacco/rch_data/health_consequences.

Centers for Disease Control. 2002 No leisure time physical activity. Behavioral risk factor surveillance system. http://apps.nccd.cdc.gov/brfss/Trends.

Chappell, N. 1992. *Social support and aging.* Toronto: Butterworths.

Chappell, N., and B. Havens. 1980. Old and female: Testing the double jeopardy hypothesis. *Sociological Quarterly* 21:157–171.

Chappell, N., E. Gee, L. McDonald, and M. Stones. 2003. *Aging in contemporary Canada.* Toronto: Prentice Hall.

Chen, J., and W. Millar. 1999. Health effects of physical activity. *Health Reports* 11:21–30.

Chen, J., and W. Millar. 2000. Are recent cohorts healthier than their predecessors? *Health Reports* 11:9–23.

Chen, J., and W. Millar. 2001a. Heart disease, family history and physical activity. *Health Reports* 12:23–32.

Chen, J., and W. Millar. 2001b. Starting and sustaining physical activity. *Health Reports* 12:33–43.

Chen, J., E. Ng, and R. Wilkins. 1996. The health of Canada's immigrants in 1994–95. *Health Reports* 7(4):33–45.

Chen, J., R. Wilkins, and E. Ng. 1996. Health expectancy by immigration status, 1986 and 1991. *Health Reports* 8(3):29–38.

CIHR. Investing in Canada's future: CIHR's blueprint for health research and innovation, Canadian Institutes of Health Research. http://www.cihr-irsc.gc.ca/about_cihr/organization/draft_corporate_plan_e.shtml.

Clark, D. O. 1996. Age, socioeconomic status, and exercise self-efficacy. *The Gerontologist* 36(2):157–64.

Clark, N., M. Becker, N. Janz, K. Lorig, W. Rakowski, and L. Anderson. 1991. Self-management of chronic disease by older adults: A review and questions for research. *Journal of Aging and Health* 3(1):3–27.

Cockerham, W., G. Lueschen, G. Kunz, and J.L. Spaeth. 1986. Social stratification and self-management of health. *Journal of Health and Social Behavior* 27:1–14.

Cole, C., and N. Castellano. 1996. *Consumer behaviour. Encyclopaedia of gerontology: Age, aging and the aged.* San Diego: Academic Press.

Coleman, J. S. 1988. Social capital in the creation of human capital. *American Journal of Sociology* 94(suppl.):S95–S120.

Courneya, K. S. 1995. Understanding readiness for regular physical activity in older individuals: An application of the theory of planned behavior. *Health Psychology* 14(1):80–87.

Crimmins, E. 1996. Mixed trends in population health among older adults. *Journal of Gerontology* 51B:S223–S225.

Crimmins, E., and Y. Saito. 2001. Trends in life expectancy in the United States, 1970–1990: Gender, racial and educational differences. *Social Sciences and Medicine* 52:1629–1641.

Curtis, J., P. White, and B. McPherson. 2000. Age and physical activity among Canadian women and men: Findings from longitudinal national survey data. *Journal of Aging and Physical Activity* 8(1): 1–20.

Day, L. 2001. The relationship between residential school attendance and health status in later life among First Nation elders in B.C. Gerontology MA Project. Simon Fraser University, Burnaby, B.C.

Denton, F.T., and B. Spencer. 1997. Population aging and the maintenance of social support systems. *Canadian Journal on Aging* 16(3):485–498.

Denton, F.T., and B. Spencer. 2000. Population aging and its economic costs: A survey of the issues and evidence. *Canadian Journal on Aging* 19(suppl. 1):1–31.

Didelez, V, I. Pigeot, K. Dean, and A.V. Wister. 2002. A comparative analysis of graphical interaction and logistic regression modelling: Self-care and coping with a chronic illness in later life. *Biometrical Journal* 44:410–432.

DiPietro, L. 2001. Physical activity in aging: Changes in patterns and their relationship to health and function. *Journals of Gerontology* 56A (series A):13–22.

Dishman, R., and J. Buckworth. 1996. Increasing physical activity. A quantitative synthesis. *Medicine and Science in Sports and Exercise* 28:706–719.

Dunn, A., R. Anderson, and J. Jakicic. 1998. Lifestyle physical activity interventions: History, short- and long-term effects, and recommendations. *American Journal of Preventive Medicine* 15:398–412.

Dunn, I., and J.R. Dyck. 2000. Social determinants of health in Canada's immigrant population: Results from the National Population Health Survey. *Social Science and Medicine* 51:1573–1593.

Dunn, J., and M. Hayes. 2000. Social inequality, population health, and housing: A study of two Vancouver neighborhoods. *Social Science and Medicine* 51:563–587.

Dychtwald, K. 1997. Wake-up call: The 10 physical, social, spiritual, economic and political crises the boomers will face as they age in the 21st century. *Critical Issues in Aging* 1:11–13.

Easterlin, R. 1991. The economic impact of prospective population changes in advanced industrial countries: A historical perspective. *Journal of Gerontology: Social Sciences* 46(6): S299–S309.

Easterlin, R. 1996. Economic and social implications of demographic patterns. In *Handbook of aging and the social sciences.* 4th ed. Edited by R. Binstock and L. George, 73– 93. San Diego: Academic Press

Eckardt, M., T. Harford, E. Koelber, S. Parker, L. Rosenthal, R. Ryback, G. Salmoiraghi, E. Vanderveen, and D. Warren. 1981. Health hazards associated with alcohol consumption. *Journal of the American Medical Association* 246:658–666.

Edwards, D. 1995. *Introduction to graphical models.* New York: Springer.

Elder, G., and R. Rockwell. 1979. Economic depression and post-war opportunity in men's lives: A study of life patterns and mental health. In *Research in community and mental health,* edited by R.G. Simmons. Greenwich, CT: JAI Press.

Evans, R., K. McGrail, S. Morgan, M. Barer, and C. Hertzman. 2001. Apocalypse no: Population aging and the future of the health care systems. *Canadian Journal on Aging* 20(suppl. 1):160–191.

Federal, Provincial and Territorial Advisory Committee on Population Health. 1999. *Toward a healthy future: Second report on the health of Canadians.* Ottawa: Minister of Public Works and Government Services Canada.

Federal, Provincial and Territorial Ministers of Health. 2003. *The integrated pan-Canadian health living strategy: A discussion document for the healthy living symposium.* Ottawa: Minister of Public Works and Government Services Canada.

Fishbein, M., and I. Ajzen. 1975. *Belief, attitude, intention, and behaviour: An intro-duction to theory and research.* Reading, MA: Addison-Wesley.

Foot, D. 1996. *Boom, bust and echo: How to profit from the coming demographic shift.* Toronto: Macfarlane Walter and Ross.

Foss, K. 2000. Famed fitness agency faces budget trimming. *Times Colonist,* 25 November.

Frankel, B., M. Speechley, and T. Wade. 1996. *The sociology of health and health care: A Canadian perspective.* Toronto: Copp Clark.

Fries, J.F. 1983. Compression of morbidity. *Milbank Memorial Fund Quarterly* 61:397–419.

Frontera, W.R., and C.N. Meredith. 1989. Strength training in the elderly. In *Physical activity, aging and sports,* edited by R. Harris and S. Harris, 319–331. Albany: Center for the Study of Aging.

Garland, C., E. Barett-Connor, L. Suarez, M.H. Criqui, and D.L. Wingard. 1985. Effects of passive smoking on ischemic heart disease mortality of non-smokers. *American Journal of Epidemiology* 121:645–650.

Gauvin, L., J. Spence, and S. Anderson. 1999. Exercise and psychological well-being in the adult population: Reality or wishful thinking? In *Textbook of medicine, exercise, nutrition and health,* edited by J. Rippe, 957–966. Malden, MA: Blackwell Publishing.

Gee, E. 2000. Voodoo demography, population aging, and social policy. In *The overselling of population aging: Apocalyptic demography, intergenerational challenges, and social policy,* edited by E. Gee and G.M. Gutman, 5–25. Don Mills, ON: Oxford University Press.

Gee, E., and G.M. Gutman, eds. 2000. *The overselling of population aging: Apocalyptic demography, intergenerational challenges, and social policy.* Don Mills, ON: Oxford University Press.

Gee, M., K. Kobayashi, and S. Prus. 2004. Examining the healthy immigrant effect in mid- to later life: Findings from the Canadian Community Health Survey. *Canadian Journal on Aging* 23 (suppl.):S55–S63.

Giele, J., and G. Elder. 1998. Life course research: Development of a field. In *Methods of life course research: Qualitative and quantitative approaches,* edited by J. Giele and G. Elder, 5–28. London: Sage.

Giele, J., and G. Elder, eds. 1998. *Methods of life course research: Qualitative and quantitative approaches.* London: Sage.

Gillman, M., B. Pinto, S. Tennstedt, K. Glanz, B. Marcus, and M. Friedman. 2001. Relationships of physical activity with dietary behaviors among adults. *Preventive Medicine* 32:295–301.

Gilmore, H., and J. Gentleman. 1999. Mortality in metropolitan areas. *Health Reports* 11(1):9–19.

Gilmore, J. 1999. Body mass index and health. *Health Reports* 11(1):31–43.

Glasgow, R.E., S. Boles, H. McKay, E. Feil, and M. Barrera. 2003. The D-Net diabetes self-management program: Long-term implementation, outcomes, and generalization results. *Preventive Medicine* 36:410–419.

Glenn, N.D. 1977. *Cohort analyses*. Beverly Hills: Sage.

Glenn, N.D. 1989. A flawed approach to solving the identification problem in the estimation of the mobility effects model: A comment by Brody and McRae. *Social Forces* 67:789–795.

Godin, G. 1994. Theories of reasoned action and planned behaviour: Usefulness for exercise promotion. *Medicine and Science in Sports and Exercise* 26(11):1391–1394.

Gottlieb, B.H. 2000. Self-help, mutual aid, and support groups among older adults. *Canadian Journal on Aging* 19(suppl. 1):58–74.

Green, L. 1980. *Health education planning: A diagnostic approach*. Baltimore: Mayfield Publishing.

Grundy, S. 1999. Primary prevention of coronary heart disease: Integrating risk assessment with intervention. *Circulation* 100:988–998.

Gutman, G.M. and A.V. Wister, eds. 1994. *Health promotion for older Canadians: Knowledge gaps and research needs*. Vancouver: Gerontology Research Centre.

Haapanen, N., S. Miilunpalo, I. Vuori, P. Oja, and M. Pasanen. 1997. Association of leisure time physical activity with the risk of coronary heart disease, hypertension and diabetes in middle-aged men and women. *International Journal of Epidemiology* 26:739–747.

Harris, D., and S. Guten. 1979. Health protective behaviour: An exploratory study. *Journal of Health and Social Behavior* 20:17–29.

Health Canada. 1993. *Canada's health promotion survey: Technical report*. Cat. H39-263/2-1990E. Ottawa: Minister of Supply and Services Canada.

Health Canada. 1994. *Strategies for population health: Investigating the health of Canadians*. Ottawa: Minister of Supply and Services Canada.

Health Canada. 1995. *Report card on the health of Canadians: Technical version*. Federal/Provincial/Territorial Advisory Committee on Population Health. Ottawa: Minister of Supply and Services Canada.

Health Canada 1998a. *Economic burden of illness, 1998*. Ottawa: Minister of Public Works and Government Services Canada.

Health Canada 1998b. *Canada's Physical Activity Guide to Healthy Active Living*. Ottawa: Minister of Public Works and Government Services Canada.

Health Canada 1998c. *Handbook for Canada's Physical Activity Guide to Healthy Active Living for Older Adults*. Ottawa: Minister of Public Works and Government Services Canada.

Health Canada. 2002. Tobacco/Smoking Website. Retrieved 13 April 2003, from http://www.hc-sc.gc.ca/hecs-sesc/tobacco/facts.

Health and Welfare Canada. 1988. *Canada's health promotion survey: Technical report.* Cat. H39–119/1988E. Ottawa: Minister of Supply and Services Canada.

Heart and Stroke Foundation of British Columbia and Yukon. 1996. Wake up call to Canadian baby boomers. *News From the Heart.* Vancouver: Heart and Stroke Foundation of British Columbia and Yukon.

Hertzman, C. 1998. The case for child development as a determinant of health. *Canadian Journal of Public Health* 89(suppl. 1):S14–S19.

Hickey, T., F. Wolf, L. Robins, M. Wagner, and W. Harik. 1995. Physical activity training for functional mobility in older persons. *Journal of Applied Gerontology* 14(4):357–371.

Hu, F. 2003. The Mediterranean diet and mortality – olive oil and beyond. *New England Journal of Medicine* 348:2595–2596.

Hu, F., E. Rimm, M. Stampfer, A. Ascherio, D. Spiegelmann, and W. Willet. 2000. Prospective study of major dietary patterns and risk of coronary heart disease in men. *American Journal of Clinical Nutrition* 72:912–921.

Human Genome Project Information. 2003. The Human Genome Project. http://www.ornl.gov/TechResources/HumanGenome.

International Longevity Centre. 2000. *Maintaining healthy lifestyles: A lifetime of choices.* A report sponsored by the International Longevity Centre, NY, USA; Canyon Ranch Health Resort; and The International Life Sciences Institute. New York: International Longevity Center.

James, R., T. Young, C. Mustard, and J. Blanchard. 1997. The health of Canadians with diabetes. *Health Reports* 9(3):47–52.

Jeffery, R., and S. French. 1998. Epidemic obesity in the United States: Are fast foods and television viewing contributing? *American Journal of Public Health* 88:277–280.

Jenkins, D., D. Popovich, C. Kendall, E. Vidgen, N. Tariq, T. Ransom, T. Wolever, V. Vuksan, C. Mehling, D. Boctor, C. Bolognesi, J. Huang, and R. Patten. 1997. Effect of a diet high in vegetables, fruit, and nuts on serum lipids. *Metabolism* 46:530–537.

Jenkins, É., Y. Carrière, and J. Légaré. 1997. Les changements qualitatifs dans le processus de renouvellement des générations: Impacts sur la mesure et la projection du besoin d'aide des personnes âgées. *Canadian Journal on Aging/Revue Canadienne du Vieillissement* 16(2):237–253.

Joffres, M.R., and D.R. MacLean.1999. Comparison of the prevalence of cardiovascular risk factors between Quebec and other Canadian provinces: The Canadian heart health surveys. *Ethnicity and Disease* 9:246–253.

Johansen, H., M. Nargundkar, C. Nair, G. Taylor, and S. ElSaadany. 1998. At risk of first or recurring heart disease. *Health Reports* 9(4):19–29.

Kaplan, M., J. Newsom, B. McFarland, and L. Lu. 2001. Demographic and psychosocial correlates of physical activity in late life. *American Journal of Preventive Medicine* 21(4):306–312.

Katzmarzyk, P. 2001. *How active are we? Summary of proceedings: A national dialogue on healthy body weights.* Ottawa: Canadian Institutes of Health research and Obesity Canada.

Katzmarzyk, P., N. Gledhill, and R. Shephard. 2000. The economic burden of physical inactivity in Canada. *Canadian Medical Association Journal* 163:1435–1440.

Kahn, R.L., and T.C. Antonucci. 1980. Convoys over the life course: Attachment, roles and social support. In *Life-span development and behaviour,* edited by P.B. Baltes and O. Brim, 253–286. New York: Academic Press.

Kendall, O., T. Lipskie, and S. MacEachern. 1997. Canadian health surveys, 1950–1997. *Chronic Diseases in Canada* 18(2):70–89.

Kendall, P. 2000. Portion distortion: Do you want that super-sized? *Nutrition News.* http://www.ext.colostate.edu/PUBS/COLUMNN/nn001010.htm.

King, A.C., J. Rejeski, and D. Buchner. 1998. Physical activity targeting older adults: A critical review. *American Journal of Preventive Medicine* 15:316–333.

Kirkey, S. 2003. Pill said to cut strokes, heart attacks by 80%. *Vancouver Sun,* 27 June.

Krick, J., and J. Sobal. 1990. Relationships between health protective behaviours. *Journal of Community Health* 15:19–34.

Kromhout, D., B. Bloemberg, J. Seidell, A. Nissinen, and A. Menotti. 2001. Physical activity and dietary fibre determine population body fat levels: The seven countries study. *International Journal of Obesity* 25:301–306.

Lamarche, P. 1988. *Tobacco use. Canada's health promotion survey: Technical report* Cat. H39–119/1988E. Ottawa: Minister of Supply and Services.

Lamarche, P., and I. Rootman.1988. *Drug use. Canada's health promotion survey: Technical Report.* Cat. H39-119/1988E. Ottawa: Minister of Supply and Services.

Lalive d'Epinay, C., and J.F. Bickel. 2003. Do young-old exercisers feel better than sedentary persons? A cohort study in Switzerland. *Canadian Journal on Aging* 22(2):155–166

Lee, C. 1993. Attitudes, knowledge, and stages of change: A survey of exercise patterns in older Australian women. *Health Psychology* 12(6):476–480.

Lee, J. 2002. Beating boomeritis. *The Vancouver Sun.* 24 June 2002.

Lenert, L., R. Munoz, J. Stoddard, K. Delucchi, A. Bansod, S. Skoczen, and E. Perez-Stable. 2003. Design and pilot evaluation of an Internet smoking cessation program. *Journal of the American Medical Information Association* 10: 16–20.

Lock, J.Q., and A.V. Wister. 1992. Intentions and changes in exercise behaviour: A lifestyle perspective. *Health Promotion International* 7(3):195–208.

Lomas, J. 1998. Social capital and health: Implications for public health and epidemiology. *Social Science and Medicine* 47(9):1181–1188.

Manson, J., P. Greenland, A. LaCroix, M. Stefanick, C. Mouton, A. Oberman, M. Perri, D. Sheps, M. Pettinger, and D. Siscovick. 2002. Walking compared with vigorous exercise for the prevention of cardiovascular events in women. *New England Journal of Medicine* 347:716–725.

Manton, K.G., E. Stallard, and L. Corder. 1997. Changes in the age dependence of mortality and disability: Cohort and other determinants. *Demography* 34:135–137.

Manuel, D., and S. Schulz. 2001. *Adding years to life and life to years: Life and health expectancy in Ontario*. Toronto: Institute for Clinical Evaluation Sciences.

Marcus, B.H., B.C. Bock, and B.M. Pinto. 1997. Initiation and maintenance of exercise behavior. In *Handbook of health behavior research II: Provider determinants*, edited by D.S. Gochman. New York: Plenum Press.

Marcus, B.H., and N. Owen. 1992. Motivational readiness, self efficacy and decision making for exercise. *Journal of Applied Social Psychology* 22:3–16.

Marcus, B.H., V.C. Selby, R.S. Niaura, and J.S. Rossi. 1992. Self-efficacy and the stages of exercise behavior change. *Research Quarterly for Exercise and Sport* 63(1): 60–66.

Marmot, M. 1993. Changing places changing risks: The study of migrants. *Public Health Reviews* 21:185–195.

Marmot, M., M. Kogevinas, and M. Elston. 1987. Social/economic status and disease. *Annual Review of Public Health* 8:111–135.

Marshall, V. 1999. Analyzing social theories of aging. In *Handbook of Theories of Aging*, edited by V. Bengtson and W. Schaie, 434–455, New York: Springer. 434–455.

McDaniel, S. 1986. *Canada's aging population*. Toronto: Butterworths.

McDonald-Miszczak, L., A.V. Wister, and G. Gutman. 2001. Self-care among older adults: An analysis of the objective and subjective illness context. *Journal of Aging and Health* 13(1):120–145.

McGinnis, J., and W. Feoge. 1993. Actual causes of death in the United States. *Journal of the American Medical Association* 270:2207–2212.

McKay, H., D. King, E. Eakin, J. Seeley, and R. Glasgow. 2001. The Diabetes Network Internet-Based Physical Activity Intervention: A randomized pilot study. *Diabetes Care* 24: 1328–1334.

McMichael, A. 1999. Prisoners of the proximate: Loosening the constraints on epidemiology in an age of change. *American Journal of Epidemiology* 149(10): 887–897.

McPherson, B.D. 1992. *Promoting active living: Policy and program perspectives*. Paper presented at the International Workshop on Health Promotion for the Elderly. Jerusalem, Israel, 16–20 November.

McPherson, B.D. 2004. *Aging as a social process: Canadian perspectives*. Toronto: Oxford University Press.

Menec, V., L. Lix, L. MacWilliam, and R. Soodeen. 2003. Trends in the health status of older Manitobans, 1985 to 1999. Paper presented at the 32nd Scientific and Educational Meetings of the Canadian Association on Gerontology, 30 Oct. – 2 Nov. 2003, Toronto.

Millar, W. 1996. Reaching smokers with lower educational attainment. *Health Reports* 8(2):11–19.

Millar, W., and T. Stephens. 1987. Overweight and obesity in Britain, Canada, and the United States. *American Journal of Public Health* 77:38–41.

Millar, W., and T. Stephens. 1993. Social status and health risks in Canadian adults: 1985 and 1991. *Health Reports* 5(2):143–156.

Mirowsky, J., and C. Ross. 1998. Education, personal control, lifestyle and health: A human capital hypothesis. *Research on Aging* 20(4):415–449.

Mitchell, B.A. 2003. Life course theory. In *The International Encyclopedia of Marriage and Family Relationships*, 2d ed. Edited by J.J. Ponzetti, 1051–1055. New York: Macmillan Reference, USA.

Moore, E., and M. Rosenberg. 1997. Growing old in Canada: Demographic and geographic perspecitives. Statistics Canada census monograph series. Toronto: Nelson.

Morgan, D. 1998a. Introduction: The aging baby boom. *Generations* 22(1):5–9.

Morgan, D. 1998b. Facts and figures about the baby boom. *Generations* 22(1):10–15.

Nawaz, H., M.L. Adams, and D.L. Katz. 2000. Physician-patient interactions regarding diet, exercise and smoking. *Preventive Medicine* 31:652–657.

Neaton, J., and D. Wentworth. 1992. Serum cholesterol, blood pressure, cigarette smoking, and death from coronary heart disease. Overall findings and differences by age for 316,099 white men. Multiple risk factor intervention trial. *Archives of Internal Medicine* 152(1):56–64.

Nielsen, S.J., and B.M. Popkin. 2003. Patterns and trends in food portion sizes, 1977–1998. *Journal of the American Medical Association* 289:450–453.

Ockene, I., and N. Miller. 1997. Cigarette smoking, cardiovascular disease, and stroke: A statement for healthcare professionals from the American Heart Association. American Heart Association Task Force on Risk Reduction. *Circulation* 96:3243–3247.

Ory, M., and G. DeFriese, eds. 1998. *Self-care in later life: Research, program and policy perspectives*. New York: Springer.

Owram, D. 1999. *Born at the right time: A history of the baby boom generation*. Toronto: University of Toronto Press.

Oyster, N., M. Morton, and S. Linnell. 1984. Physical activity and osteoporosis in post-menopausal women. *Medicine and Science in Sports and Exercise* 16:44–50.

Paffenbarger, R.S., R.T. Hyde, and A.L. Wing. 1990. Physical activity and physical fitness as determinants of health and longevity. In *Exercise, fitness and health*, edited by C. Bouchard, R.J. Shephard, T. Stephens, J.R. Sutton, and B.D. McPherson, 33–48. Champaign, IL: Human Kinetics Publishers.

Palmore, E. (1978). When can age, period, and cohort effects be separated? *Social Forces* 57:282–295.

Pappas, G., S. Queen, W. Hadden, and G. Fisher. 1993. The increasing disparity in mortality between socio-economic groups in the United States, 1960 and 1986. *New England Journal of Medicine* 329:103–109.

Penning, M. 1983. Multiple jeopardy: Age, sex and ethnic variations. *Canadian Ethnic Studies* 15:81–105.

Perez, C. 2002a. Fruit and vegetable consumption. *Health Reports* 13:23–31.

Perez, C. 2002b. Health status and health behaviour among immigrants. *Health Reports* 13:1–12.

Physical Activity Monitor. 2000. Prevalence of physical inactivity. Canadian Fitness and Lifestyle Research Institute. http://www.CFLRI.ca.

Prochaska, J.O., and B.H. Marcus. 1994. The transtheoretical model: Applications to exercise. In *Advances in exercise adherence*, edited by R.K. Dishman, 161–180. Windsor, ON: Human Kinetics.

Prochaska, J.O., C.C. DiClemente, and J.C. Norcross. 1992. In search of how people change: Applications to addictive behaviors. *American Psychologist* 47(9):1102–1114.

Prohaska, T. 1998. The research basis for the design and implementation of self-care programs. In *Self-care in later life: Research, program and policy perspectives*, edited by M. Ory and G. DeFriese, 62–84. New York: Sage.

Rabkin, S., and Y. Chen. 1997. Risk factor correlates of body mass index. *Canadian Medical Association Journal* 157(1):S26–S32.

Rachlis, M., and C. Kushner. 1994. *Strong medicine: How to save Canada's health care system.* Toronto: HarperCollins.

Rakowski, W. 1992. Association of physical activity with mortality among older adults in the Longitudinal Study of Aging (1984–1988). *Journals of Gerontology* 47(4): M122–M129.

Raphael, D., ed. 2004. Social determinants of health: Canadian perspectives. Toronto: Canadian Scholars' Press.

Riley, M.W. 1993. A theoretical basis for research on health. In *Population health research: Linking theory and methods*, edited by K. Dean, 37–53. London: Sage.

Robert, S., and J. House. 1996. SES differentials in health by age and alternative indicators of SES. *Journal of Aging and Health* 8(3): 359–388.

Robine, J.M., P. Mormiche, and C. Sermet. 1998. Examination of the causes and mechanisms of the increase in disability-free life expectancy. *Journal of Aging and Health* 10(2):171–191.

Rogers, M.E. 2003. Lifestyle acculturation and health among older foreign-born persons. MA thesis. Simon Fraser University, Burnaby, BC.

Rosenstock, I. 1974. Historical origin of the Health Belief Model. *Health Education Monographs* 2:328–335.

Ruchlin, H. 1997. Prevalence and correlates of alcohol use among older adults. *Preventive Medicine* 26:651–657.

Ryder, N. 1965. The cohort as a conception in the study of social change. *American Sociological Review* 30(6):843–861.

Schaie, W. 1965. A general model for the study of developmental problems. *Psychological Bulletin* 64(2):92–107.

Schlosser, E. 2002. *Fast food nation*. New York: Houghton Mifflin.

Selvin, S. 1996. *Statistical analysis of epidemiologic data*. New York: Oxford University Press.

Scsso, H., R. Paffenbarger, and I.M. Lee. 2000. Physical activity and coronary heart disease in men: The Harvard alumni health study. *Circulation* 102:975–980.

Sesso, H., R. Paffenbarger, T. Ha, and I.M. Lee. 1999. Physical activity and cardiovascular disease risk in middle-aged and older women. *American Journal of Epidemiology* 150:408–416.

Shepard, R. 1987. *Physical activity and aging*. Champaign, IL: Human Kinetics Publishers.

Shepard, R., and W. Montelpare. 1988. Geriatric benefits of exercise as an adult. *Journals of Gerontology* 43(4):M86–M90.

Sherwood, N., and R. Jeffery. 2000. The behavioural determinants of exercise: Implications for physical activity interventions. *Annual Review of Nutrition* 20: 21–44.

Single, E., L. Gliksman, and J. LeCavalier. 2000. *Towards a Canadian health research institute of addictions*. Concept paper prepared on behalf of the Addictions Foundation of Manitoba, the Alberta Alcohol and Drug Abuse Commission, and the Canadian Centre on Substance Abuse.

Single, E., L. Robson, J. Rehm, and X. Xie. 1999. Morbidity and mortality attributable to alcohol, tobacco, and illicit drug use in Canada. *American Journal of Public Health* 89(3): 385–390.

Single, E., L. Robson, X. Xie, and J. Rehm. 1998. The economic costs of alcohol, tobacco and illicit drugs in Canada. *Addiction* 93:991–1006.

Skokdstam, L., L. Hagfors, and G. Johansson. 2003. An experimental study of a Mediterranean diet intervention for patients with rheumatoid arthritis. *Annals of the Rheumatic Diseases* 62:208–214.

Slater, M., M. Basil, and E. Maiback. 1999. A cluster analysis of alcohol-related attitudes and behaviors in the general population. *Journal of Studies on Alcohol* 60: 667–674.

Smith, P., and B. Torrey. 1996. The future of the behavioral and social sciences: Policy forum. *Science* 271(2):611–612.

Sobal, J., D. Revicki, and B. DeForge. 1992. Patterns of interrelationships among health-promotion behaviors. *American Journal of Preventive Medicine* 8(6):351–359.

Spence, J., R. Shephard, C. Craig, and K. McGannon. 2001. *Compilation of evidence of effective active living interventions: A case study approach*. Report submitted to Health Canada on behalf of the Canadian Consortium of Health Promotion Research. Ottawa: Health Canada.

Spirduso, W.W., and P. Gilliam-MacRae. 1991. Physical activity and quality of life in the frail elderly. In *Concept and measurement of quality of life in the frail elderly*, edited by J.E. Birren, J.E. Lubben, J.C. Rowe, and D.E. Deutchman, 226–255. San Diego: Academic Press.

Starkey, L., L. Johnson-Down, and K. Gray-Donald. 2001. Food habits of Canadians: Comparison of food intake in adults and adolescents to *Canada's food guide to healthy eating. Canadian Journal of Dietetic Practice and Research* 62:61–69.

Statistics Canada. 1995a. The health of Canadians. *The Daily*. Cat. 11-001F.

Statistics Canada. 1995b. *National population health survey overview 1994–1995.* Cat. 82-567. Ottawa: Minister of Industry.

Statistics Canada 1998a. Immigrant population by place of birth and period of immigration, 1996 Census, Canada. *Statistics Canada, 1996 Census Nation tables.* Retrieved 5 April 2002 from http://www.statcan.ca/english/Pgdb/People/Population/demo25a.htm.

Statistics Canada. 1998b. Population 15 years and over by highest level of schooling, 1976–1996 censuses, Canada. Retrieved 5 April 2002 from http://www.statcan.ca/English/Pgdb/educ45.htm.

Statistics Canada. 1999a. Health among older adults. *Health Reports* 11(3):47–61, cat. 82-003.

Statistics Canada. 1999b. Health in mid-life. *Health Reports* 11(3):35–46, cat. 82-003.

Statistics Canada. 1999c. Personal health practices: Smoking, drinking, physical activity and weight. *Health Reports* 11(3):83–90, cat. 82–003.

Statistics Canada. 2000. Television viewing. *The Daily* (fall):1–6.

Statistics Canada. 2001a. *International migrants, by age group and sex, Canada, provinces and territories.* Table 510011. CANSIM II. Series V437339.

Statistics Canada. 2001b. Working with computers. *The Daily* (23 May):1–2.

Statistics Canada. 2003. *Distribution of total income for individuals, T402. Income Trends in Canada, 1980–2001.* CANSIM II. Series 13F0022XCB.

Stokols, D. 1992. Establishing and maintaining healthy environments: Towards a social ecology of health promotion. *American Psychologist* 47(1):6–22.

Struempler, B. 2002. Fast-food meals are choice for most Americans. http://www.aces.edu/dept/extcomm/newspaper/fastfoods.htm.

Susser, M., and E. Susser. 1996a. Choosing a future for epidemiology: I. Eras and paradigms. *American Journal of Public Health* 86(5):668–673.

Susser, M., and E. Susser. 1996b. Choosing a future for epidemiology: II. From black box to Chinese boxes and eco-epidemiology. *American Journal of Public Health* 86(5):674–677.

Syme, L., and L. Berkman. 1979. Social class, susceptibility, and sickness. *American Journal of Epidemiology* 104:1–8.

Thompson, P., D. Buchner, I. Pina, G. Balady, M. Williams, et al. 2003. Exercise and physical activity in the prevention and treatment of atherosclerotic cardiovascular disease. *Circulation* 107:3109–3116.

Trovato, F. 1993. Mortality differences by nativity during 1985–87. *Canadian Studies in Population* 20: 207–224.

Tucker, L., and M. Bagwell. 1991. Television viewing and obesity in adult females. *American Journal of Public Health* 81:908–911.

Tucker, L., and G. Friedman. 1989. Television viewing and obesity in adult males. *American Journal of Public Health* 79:516–518.

U.S. Department of Health, Education and Welfare. 1979. *Smoking and health: A report of the Surgeon General*. Rockville, MD: U.S. Department of Health, Education and Welfare, Public Health Service, Office of the Assistant Secretary for Health, Office on Smoking and Health.

U.S. Department of Health and Human Services. 2000. *Reducing tobacco use: A report of the Surgeon General*. Atlanta: Department of Health and Human Services.

Weber, M. 1946. Class, status, party. In *Max Weber: Essays in sociology,* edited by H. Gerth and C.W. Mills. New York: Oxford University Press.

Weinstein, N., A. Rothman, and S. Sutton. 1998. Stage theories of health behavior: Conceptual and methodological issues. *Health Psychology* 17:290–299.

Wilkins, R., and O. Adams. 1987. Health expectancy in Canada, late 1970s. In *Health and Canadian society: Sociological perspectives*, edited by D. Coburn, C.D'Arcy, G. Torrance, and P. New, 36–56. Markham, ON: Fitzhenry and Whiteside.

Wing, R.R., M. Goldstein, K. Acton, L. Birch, J. Jakicic, J. Sallis, D. Smith-West, R. Jeffery, and R. Surwit. 2001. Behavioural science research in diabetes: Lifestyle changes related to obesity, eating behavior, and physical activity. *Diabetes Care* 24: 117–123.

Wister, A.V. 1995. The relationship between self-help group participation and other health behaviours among older adults. *Canadian Journal of Community Mental Health* 14(2):23–38.

Wister, A.V. 1996. The effects of socio-economic status on exercise and smoking: Age-related differences. *Aging and Health* 8(4):467–488.

Wister, A.V. 1999. Exercise change among older adults managing a chronic illness. Invited presentation for the International Longevity Centre Workshop Series: How to Initiate and Maintain Healthy Behaviors and Lifestyles, Canyon Ranch Health Resort, Tucson, AZ. 9–12 December 1999.

Wister, A.V. 2003. Health promotion and aging: It's never too late. Editorial. *Canadian Journal on Aging* 22(2):149–153.

Wister, A.V. 2004. Paradigm shifts in understanding healthy lifestyles and aging. Unpublished manuscript.

Wister, A.V. In press. The built environment, health and longevity: Multilevel salutogenic and pathogenic pathways. *Journal of Housing for the Elderly.*

Wister, A.V., and P.A. Dykstra. 2000. Formal support among Dutch older adults: An examination of the gendered nature of marital history. *Canadian Journal on Aging* 19(4):508–535.

Wister, A.V., and E.M. Gee. 1994. Age at death due to ischemic heart disease: Gender differences. *Social Biology* 41:110–126.

Wister, A.V., and G. Gutman. 1994. Using large data sets to study health promotion for older adults. In *Health promotion for older Canadians: Knowledge gaps and research needs*, edited by G.M. Gutman and A.V. Wister,125–143. Vancouver: Gerontology Research Centre.

Wister, A.V., and Z. Romeder. 2002 The chronic illness context in exercise self-care among older adults: A longitudinal analysis. *Canadian Journal on Aging* 21(4): 521–534.

Wister, A.V., M. Chittenden, B. McCoy, K. Wilson, T. Allen, and M. Wong. 2002. Using alternative therapies to manage chronic illness among older adults: An examination of the health context and enabling factors. *Canadian Journal on Aging* 21(1):45–59.

Wolf, A.M., and G.A. Coldita. 1994. The cost of obesity: The U.S. perspective. *Pharmoeconomics* 5:37.

Wolinsky, F.D. 1993. Age, period and cohort analyses of health related behaviour. In *Population health research: Linking theory and methods*, edited by K. Dean, 54–73. London: Sage.

World Health Organization. 1986. Life-styles and health. *Social Science and Medicine* 22:117–124.

World Health Organization. 1997. *Obesity: Preventing and managing the global epidemic*. Report of the WHO Consultation on Obesity. Geneva: World Health Organization.

World Health Organization. 2000. *Global strategy for prevention and control of non-communicable diseases: Report of the Director-General*. Geneva: World Health Organization.

Writing Group for the Activity Counseling Trial Research Group, The. 2001. Effects of physical activity counseling in primary care. *Journal of the American Medical Association* 286:677–687.

Yen, I., and S. Syme. 1999. The social environment and health: A discussion of the epidemiologic literature. *Annual Review of Public Health* 20: 287–308.

Young, A. 1986. Exercise physiology in geriatric practice. *Acta Medica Scandinavica* (suppl.):211–227.

Index